GRANDMOTHER'S
CURES

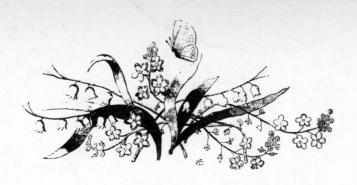

GRANDMOTHER'S CURES

& *Herbal Remedies*

DENNIS PRINCE

First published in Great Britain in 1991 by
Fontana, an imprint of HarperCollins
Publishers, 77–85 Fulham Palace Road,
Hammersmith, London W6 8JB

9 8 7 6 5 4 3 2 1

A CIP record for this book is available from
the British Library

ISBN 0 20716920 9

Printed and bound in Great Britain by
HarperCollins Book Manufacturing,
Glasgow

Contents

Acknowledgements

This book is dedicated to those wonderful 'grandmothers' of yesteryear and to their knowledge of Mother Nature's natural medications and medicines.

I would like to thank all those who sent me their stories relating to experiences of these cures, as well as my editor, Val Hudson, and publishers, HarperCollins, for without their co-operation these old remedies would surely have been lost forever.

And my thanks to Eveline Lewis who assisted me in arranging those tales, and to my wife for putting up with me while I was writing this book.

Introduction

Until comparatively recently, a visit to the doctor was an absolute last resort. Doctors were regarded with awe, distrust and suspicion and little faith was placed in the medicines prescribed, with their strange titles and unfamiliar ingredients. Far greater comfort was to be found in the remedies suggested by 'Grandma', which were homely, reassuring and in many cases, really effective. Tried and tested over the years, handed on through generations, the herbal remedies had familiar names and a proven reputation. Some may even have been designed to deter the malingerer – being so disgusting that the 'patient' was immediately and miraculously 'cured'!

It is becoming apparent however, through developments in medical research, that many of these old remedies do have a sound basis and many modern drugs use chemicals whose properties have been recognised by the analysis of plants used in herbal medicine.

You may find echoes of forgotten conversations and chance remarks in this book, perhaps awakening memories of the way things used to be done to effect a 'cure' in the days before prescribed medicines. And, you will most certainly be intrigued and entertained by these examples of 'Grandmother's Cures.'

A note from the Editor

These restoratives and remedies, concoctions and herbal cures may charm and intrigue you, but they are not recommended as treatments. *Do not* experiment with attributed medicinal properties, always consult a trained herbalist, doctor or physician.

The Publishers and Author accept no responsibility for any adverse effects directly or indirectly resulting from the use of 'Grandmother's Cures & Herbal Remedies.'

PART ONE

A TO Z OF CURES

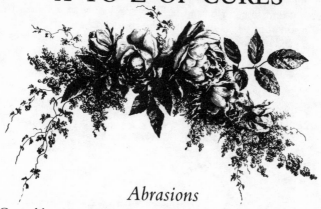

Abrasions

Caused by scratching or any other breaking of the skin. One must first ensure the sore is thoroughly cleansed of dirt or grit. Bathe with boracic lotion then apply iodine.

Abscess

Take from the garden a large parsnip, boil to pulp consistency and strain. Bathe the affected part with strained water, then apply the parsnip pulp as hot as can be borne.

Take some lily of the valley leaves, steep in boiling water. Put into muslin then apply as a poultice. Bandage and leave overnight. Repeat until cure is effected.

To cure make a poultice of monkey musk flower and hot water, place on the abscess and secure by bandaging.

Acidity (of the Stomach)

Symptoms such as heartburn, flushing of the face and many other disagreeable feelings accompany this disorder. To relieve one must first contain the acidity. This is best done by taking two teaspoons of magnesia in a tumbler of milk or half a teaspoon of bicarbonate of soda in reasonably hot water.

Acne or Adolescent Spots

One cupful of nettle tea night and morning, made by boiling nettles for two hours and decanting liquid. The nettles can also be eaten as a vegetable.

To get rid of ugly spots, after washing take the leaf of the iceplant and break a piece off, then rub the open ends of the leaf upon spots. In a short time the spots will disappear. Also good used in the same way to heal cuts, grazes and cold sores.

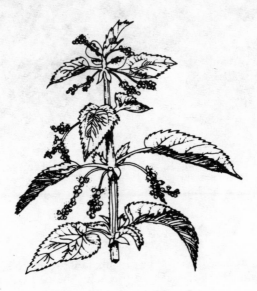

Adenoids

To relieve, the sufferer should sniff into their nose salted water.

Ageing

To allay ageing one should take of the 'Miracle Brew'. To make: gather a handful of healthy stinging nettles, dandelion flowers and roots and some red clover. Stew in two pints of water for two hours, strain liquid, add sugar and honey, juice of three lemons and a spoonful of liquid yeast. Leave overnight, next morning strain and bottle. Works marvels. Is also said to stop one going bald.

Asthma

Should one suffer this complaint one would be ill advised to eat a large meal before going to bed. Foodstuffs known to aggravate this condition are pork, cheese and pastry. A warm glass of milk drunk by the patient whilst in bed, in many cases will ward off an attack. Herbal tobacco, of which half should be 'coltsfoot', smoked in a pipe will also relieve this condition.

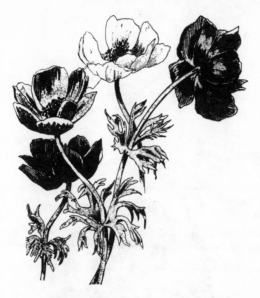

Backache and Hip Pains

Stand with feet about eighteen inches apart, place palms of hands on hips, then lean back alternating from the left and right. To relieve aching hips sit on the floor, open your legs approximately four feet, place both hands first onto your left leg, then push forward as far as possible, repeat four or five times, and then do same on the right leg. The pain will go. Repeat if pain returns.

Back (Weak)

Massage using methylated spirits, after which the back should be dusted with starch powder. This is most soothing and cool.

Baldness

It is thought that dandruff is one of the main causes of premature baldness. To contain the loss of hair the head should be washed at least once a week with soap and soft water, the scalp should be massaged with a concoction of three parts of almond oil to one of spirits or wine. A lotion of a tablespoon of flowers of sulphur shaken up in a bottle of water, rubbed into the scalp, will keep it free of dandruff.

Bed Sores

The parts taking the weight should be constantly changed, these should also be sponged each day after bathing with equal parts of methylated spirits and oil, and then dusted with starch powder.

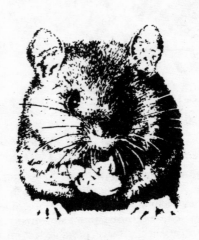

Bedwetting

The child who wets the bed should be fed unknown a boiled or fried field mouse. After which bedwetting will stop.

Biliousness

When suffering this complaint no food should be taken, a full day's fast is recommended and where possible one is advised to take to bed for complete rest. The stomach should be purged of any undigested matter. The stomach should also be thoroughly washed by drinking large amounts of water, or soda water.

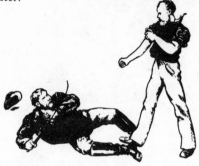

Black Eye

Take a little bicarbonate of soda, add to hot water. This solution when used to bathe eye brings relief.

Bladder (Inflammation and Cystitis)

Symptoms: pain in the small of the back, frequent passing of water, strong smell to urine. The mixture for relief is 15 grains of citrate of potash, ½ oz. infusion of buchu.★ The patient should stay in bed, have hot fomentations, take only a simple diet, and drink ample barley water.

Bleeding Nose

To stop one should sniff or snuffle into offending nostril powdered alum.

In full blooded persons slight bleeding of the nose may be beneficial, it often gives relief to headache. If severe, cold water should be applied to the nose and nape of the neck, and the nose held between forefinger and thumb. If this does not arrest it, a handkerchief should be torn into strips and used to plug the nose, continuing the bathing with cold water. (Do not lie patient on their back.)

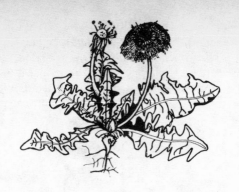

Blood Impurities

To rid the blood of impurities infuse dandelion and worm-wood, strain and bottle liquid, take a small wineglass full each morning.

To purify one should mix sulphur with home rendered lard.

Also take spoonful of brimstone and treacle.

Bloodlessness (Anaemia)

A condition suffered most frequently by young women. Lack of colour and palpitations are usual giveway signs to a sufferer of this condition. The patient should take only of easily digested foods, they should also rest both bodily and mentally. Constipation usually accompanies this complaint. This can be relieved by taking a dose of salt in water each morning before breakfast. Iron must be taken into the system, one to three aloes and iron pills three times a day after food.

Blood Poisoning (Arm or Leg)

To cure mix some fine oatmeal with cold milk to a stiff paste – a bit thicker than one mixes mustard – and apply this on a clean piece of linen, make sure it is large enough to cover all cuts and bind up. Leave on overnight. As plaster hardens it will draw poison from limb.

Boils

Use a bread poultice to draw out pus and relieve soreness. Scald a piece of white bread, squeeze out water, wrap in linen and place on boil.

From the gunsmith buy as much gunpowder as would cover a sixpenny piece. Roll it in a piece of butter and make a pill of it, this should then be swallowed. In a very short time the boils will clear up.

This cure should only be used when boil is ripe. Fill bottle with hot water, leave water in bottle until glass is heated right through, tip out water and immediately place neck of bottle on boil. The suction and heat will cause the boil to burst. This method ensures that the core of the boil is removed.

'Fiddler's Rosit' (powdered resin), the dosage being the amount which can be carried on a silver threepenny piece, mixed with jam to help it down. This to be taken once or twice a day until the condition shows signs of improvement. It is important to take Rosit only when one has boils.

Bathe boils with hot salt water, as hot as can be borne.

To rid oneself of boils grind a nutmeg to powder, mix with a little water and consume.

Eat one large raw Spanish onion.

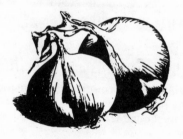

Breath

For offensive breath through stomach disorders, take six drops of concentrated solution of common salt in a glass of water first thing in the morning. Should the cause be decayed teeth, the mouth should be well rinsed using one teaspoon of salt in a tumbler of warm water. For breath smelling of garlic or onions, eat a few leaves of parsley after dipping them in vinegar.

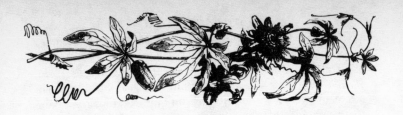

Bronchitis

The sufferer should take to bed or keep to a warm room. Attacks of bronchitis can be relieved in a few days if the patient follows this simple advice. The bowels should be kept open. Hot milk will loosen the phlegm. Mustard poultices should be applied to chest, or rub with hartshorn and oil. Children should be given hot home-made lemonade at bed-time. If they are having difficulty with sleeping: add to the lemonade one or two tablespoons of whisky. For adults, take a jug of steaming water, add a teaspoon of Friar's Balsam or a few drops of eucalyptus oil, place a towel over the patient's head. The vapour should then be breathed in deeply. Ensure the eyes are kept closed.

To a basinful of boiling water add one teaspoonful each of oils of camphor, eucalyptus and menthol. Mix well. Cover head and shoulders with a large towel and breathe deeply of fumes given off. Top up occasionally with hot water and the mucous membranes and bronchial tubes will clear.

Bruises, Sprains and Swellings

Bathe with an infusion of comfrey leaves made by stewing the leaves gently for two hours at low heat. Bandage a sprain using a few of the boiled leaves next to the skin.

Bunions

A simple treatment for bunions is to treat it with solution made from comfrey powder or root, this can be obtained from any herbalist. Two tablespoonfuls mixed in one pint of water, brought slowly to the boil, simmered for half an hour and then strained into a basin. A pint is enough to enable three soakings of the foot and three-quarters of that mixture is sufficient bathing water.

Burns and Scalds

If the burn is slight and the part is red and blistered, flour or ground starch should be dusted lavishly upon it to exclude air. Lanolin or castor oil will answer the same purpose. The burn should then be protected from further injury by covering with clean hanky or piece of lint. When the burns are of a deep nature, the clothes must be removed carefully. The burn then bathed in Condy's fluid, boracic acid or any antiseptic, then lint smeared with boracic ointment applied. The patient should be put to bed, hot water bottles to feet, then given stimulants or strong tea or coffee.

To alleviate pain pour white of egg over wound, this will also prevent inflammation.

To relieve and aid healing of burns rub immediately and liberally with goose grease.

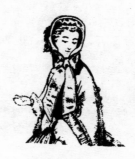

(From Acids)

Wash immediately with limewater, carbonate of soda and water, whiting and water or chalk and water. Then apply the mixture of chalk and oil (see following entry). For burns from sulphuric acid, bathe with linseed oil for ten minutes.

(From Lime)

Bathe with vinegar and water, dress with chalk that has been mixed to a thin paste with linseed oil. Renew the treatment at intervals.

(Minor)

To ease pain rub gently with sliced raw potato.

Camomile Tea

To make: Drop ½oz camomile flowers into 1 pint of boiling water, simmer for 15 minutes, then strain. When warm it may be used as an emetic, taken when cold is a good tonic.

Carbuncles

Carbuncles start as a hard tender swelling. The skin becomes inflamed and hot, then it blisters. These eventually burst and allow the contents of the carbuncle to discharge. Treatment: take of good food and a fair amount of stimulants. A teaspoonful of Parrish's food in water should be taken three times a day after meals. The affected part should be washed constantly.

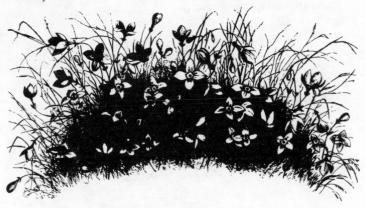

Catarrh

This is an inflammation of the mucous membrane, and affects both the head and throat. The best time for treatment of this condition is in the warm summer months. In chronic cases a little boracic acid powder should be snuffed up the nostrils. This will attack and kill the germs and so prepare the way for the following, which has both soothing and healing properties, to be used in an atomizer. Mix together 12 drops of sandalwood oil, 15 drops of wintergreen, 8 drops of oil cassia or cinnamon, 15 grains of menthol and 4oz medoline. Use night and morning. Another form of treatment that is very effective: one teaspoon of common salt stirred into a cup of warm water, this solution to be snuffed up nose at bedtime and morning.

Chest Complaints

The sufferer should be taken, early in the morning, to a field where there are cows. When a cow rises from its night's sleep the sufferer should immediately lie in the warm spot vacated by the cow.

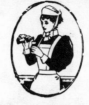

Chicken Pox

Symptoms: Child feels ill; within twenty-four hours small pimples form on the scalp, neck, back, chest and shoulders but these rarely erupt on face. On the third day these mature and slowly fade – others making their appearance at the same time. Chicken pox although not dangerous, is very infectious. The quarantine time is three weeks; the child after infection will almost certainly be left in a weak state, and so should be given a tonic, fresh air and good food.

Colds

(To Ward Off)

Wear a square of camphor in a small bag around the neck from November to May. Replace camphor as it wastes away.

(Cures)

Take a sock that has been worn, place around patient's neck on going to bed. Smelly but successful.

Elder blossom. Pick it at a tender young stage, hang it in bunches, leave to dry. Steep in boiling water. Must be drunk very hot if suffering a persistent cold. Also very good for persistent coughs.

Take one tot of whisky while resting feet in mustard foot-bath. A very acceptable cure.

After a hot bath, Russian tallow spread thickly on brown paper should be plastered on chest. A remedy used to cure many complaints (Chest or Bronchial).

Corns

To remove the hard cuticle which forms the corn, soak the feet for half an hour on two or three nights in a strong solution of soda.

Soak an ivy leaf in vinegar and apply to corn. This should do the trick.

To cure stand a piece of potash in the open air until it powders then mix to a paste with powdered gum arabic. Apply to affected part.

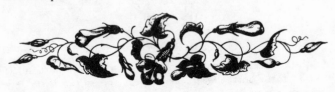

Coughs

Chop a good quantity of parsley and mix it with a little hot milk (do not cook parsley) the mixture should be thick. Sup it down then retire from society to cough up loosened phlegm (Bronchial cough).

Make a strong solution of saltpetre dissolved in water. Get a clean sheet of white blotting paper, thoroughly soak this sheet in the saltpetre solution then allow to dry. Cut off a corner and place in a saucer, set fire to edge (it will burn like touch paper) let the patient inhale the smoke, hold the mouth open over the saucer and draw fumes in. It should be done sitting up in bed last thing. White blotting paper is named because there is nothing injurious in the making thereof.

Into a dish put layers of turnips, sliced. Sprinkle each layer with brown sugar, leave for twelve hours. The syrup formed should be taken whenever needed.

Slice a large onion into layers. Place bottom layer into a basin then cover with brown sugar. Repeat this with each layer until onion is whole again; leave overnight. The syrup that will form is very good for those suffering with bad chest colds, especially children, and may be taken any time of the day.

Take the white of an egg, to this add a pinch of salt, whip to a froth. A spoonful to be taken three or four times at hourly intervals.

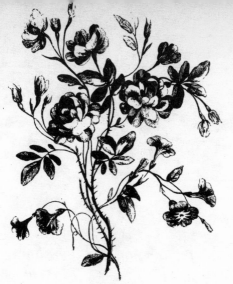

Cough Mixture

Mix together 4oz honey, 1 gill vinegar, 4oz golden syrup and 2 paregoric. Take one spoonful three times a day, or whenever cough is troublesome.

Cramp

Rub affected part with a piece of cork.

(Night Cramp)

Keep a lump of sulphur at the foot of the bed and when you get an attack place your foot onto the sulphur.

Cuts

No cut should ever be neglected no matter how small. The cut should first be sucked and then placed beneath tap, after which it should be bathed in Condy's fluid, or other antiseptic. Friar's Balsam will stop bleeding.

Dandruff

To prevent, rub raw egg into scalp when washing hair.

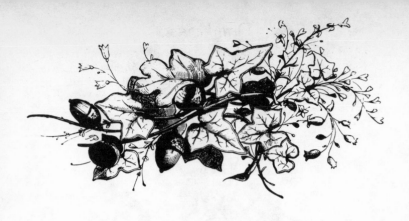

Depression and Tension

To relieve, lie down and place hot water bottle on kneecaps.

Diarrhoea

Take as much tincture of red lavender as can be absorbed on a lump of sugar. Tincture of red lavender can only be obtained from very old fashioned chemists.

Take of finely grated acorns.

Sometimes caused by change of diet or conflicting foodstuffs causing irritation in bowels. Try first two teaspoonsful of castor oil to remove irritant. If still persisting, take about six iron pills, one each at hourly intervals. Alternatively use spinach as vegetable for several meals.

Diptheria

Steep elderflowers (fresh or dried flowers will do) in water. Bathe the neck with the solution, also take a few teaspoonsful to drink if possible.

Dropsy

Cut young shoots of gorse bush, boil in water for fifteen minutes. Give patient liquid.

Drunkenness

To cure: take 5 grains sulphate of iron, 10 grains magnesia, 11 drams peppermint water, 1 dram spirits of nutmeg. This acts as a tonic, is also a stimulant and so partly takes the place of liquor the patient would normally crave. It also helps counteract withdrawal symptoms. Start by giving the patient twelve drops on a lump of sugar, then increase till two teaspoons of concoction are taken twice a day.

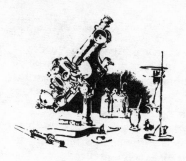

Earache

Put a moderate amount of salt into a clean cloth. Warm in oven then place under ear. Retain overnight, in the morning the ear will have discharged all pus and rubbish and will be easy.

Drop a small amount of olive oil into ear and rub underneath with camphor oil.

Place index fingers half an inch below each ear, press gently and you will find this will gently ease the pain away until eventually it goes completely. (Also good for headache and toothache.)

Break the leaf of the iceplant, squeeze the sap onto warmed saucer, spoon into ear.

Heat large onion, squeeze the juice from it. When cool spoon juice into offending ear.

Place a small plug of cotton wool dipped into warmed almond oil in the affected ear.

The ear should be gently rinsed using warm water; to ease apply hot flannel to side of head. Another form of ease is to place mustard leaf behind ear. One must not tamper inside ear.

Eczema (and Skin Irritation)

To relieve this condition, collect and thoroughly wash a large handful of watercress. Put into pan, cover with water. Bring to the boil then simmer until all goodness is extracted and the shoots are tender. Strain liquid through muslin and allow to cool. Bathe affected area two to three times a day using clean cloth for each wash. This is also effective in treating skin chafed and sore by wind. Soap should not be used on either of these conditions.

Collect an armful of chickweed, wash well and place in a bucket, pour on enough boiling water to just cover, leave overnight. Next day press chickweed down with tongs or potato masher and then strain water through colander, let it settle, then strain through muslin or tea towel. Bottle and keep in fridge, apply as needed to affected parts. (Also cure for ringworm.)

Dig up some burdock roots and stew them, strain off the water. Drink a small wineglass full every morning for nine days, leave for nine days and then repeat, continue treatment for three months. A very effective cure.

To cure, put small quantity of crystals of Condy's fluid into the bath water, which will turn water red.

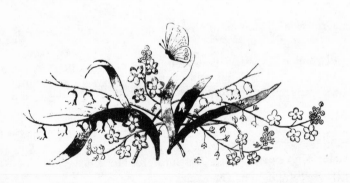

Emetics

To explain simply these are used to promote vomiting. In case of poisoning they should be given immediately. Strong salt in water, or strong mustard in water. They should never be given in cases of burning poisons.

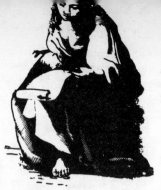

Eye and Eyelids (Inflamed)

Should you suffer this, bathe with lukewarm water and Condy's fluid.

'Eyewater' a dilute solution of zinc sulphate, dropped into the eye from a teaspoon.

Eye Trouble

To relieve, bathe with an infusion of the herb eyebright, or dissolve a pinch of boracic acid crystals in half a teacupful of water and use in eyeglass, after cooling liquid.

Feet

(Aching)

To take the burning from feet when walking, place within the shoes a dock leaf, smooth side up.

Most suffer this at some time. To ease hot or aching feet, boil a quart of bran in one and a half gallons of water for five minutes. Leave to cool enough to immerse feet, soak until water is lukewarm.

Mix two tablespoons of mustard to a paste adding a little cold water, this to be added to bath as drawn.

(Blistered)

To relieve this, change socks left to right and vice-versa after rubbing soles of socks with dry soap. Where blistering occurs treat with boracic ointment.

(Bunions)

Purchase a bottle of meatsfoot oil from chemist's shop, rub on the bunion night and morning. The bunion will gradually shrink and disappear.

(Chilblains)

Soak feet in cold urine.

'Thrash' with fresh holly branches. Drastic but most effective.

Make a paste of baking soda and apply to the affected part.

Dissolve six pearl buttons in the juice of one lemon. Apply to chilblains.

(Chilblains – to prevent)

Sprinkle grated onion into socks.

(Cold)

Sprinkle a little powdered mustard into socks.

Before going out on a freezing night shake a good layer of pepper into shoes.

(Corns)

Pluck the flowers of the elder tree on a fine day and spread them on a newspaper to dry. Store them in paper bags. Two handfuls in water and soak corns, corns will soon be cured.

To cure soak an ivy leaf in vinegar and apply to corn. This will bring instant relief.

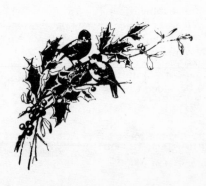

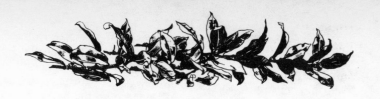

(Corns – to prevent)

Zinc and castor oil ointment rubbed into feet daily prevents corns.

(Sore Heel)

Take leaves of the white lily, place on heels and bandage in place. Heels should be cured within two days.

(Sweaty)

Damp down a small quantity of bran and rub onto feet ensuring it is pressed between the toes.

One should bathe feet if they smell in one of the following solutions every night:
Plenty of borax and water.
A pinch of permanganate of potash in eight ounces of water.
Tablespoon of common soda in a quart of water.
Dry thoroughly, powder with chalk.

(Tender)

Sponge feet morning and night with solution of carbonate of soda and water or salt and water, mixed two tablespoons to one pint.

(Tired)

Bathe in two quarts of water as hot as one can bear, add to this a handful of salt. This will stimulate the circulation and remove the waste products that are responsible for the fatigue. Two handfuls of salt to a basin of hot water.

Take lily of the valley leaves, place in the bottom of shoes or boots, wear during day.

(Verruca)

Take a knob of soda, rub on verruca night and morning. Within a few days the verruca will disappear.

Fever

(To Break)

From the butcher's buy two melts. They are like pieces of liver, they must be fresh. Tie to bottom of the patient's feet, they will then draw the fever and bring down the patient's temperature if left overnight.

Gather a large number of earthworms and fill a man's woollen sock with them. The sock should then be put around the patient's neck and left overnight. In the morning the patient will be cool and the worms will have dissolved into oil.

Steep elderberry flowers in boiling water, give liquid to patient.

(Rheumatic)

Grate salt from block enough to cover the bottom of a large roasting dish, place in oven to warm. Place enough amounts in a pair of socks and place on feet of sufferer, this to be done three times daily. This remedy should show results in a week.

(Scarlet)

Soak gauze squares in camphor oil, place in brassière or vest.

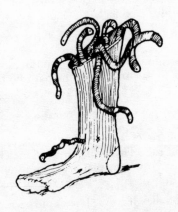

Fits

Half fill a bath with tepid water, pour in half tin of mustard powder. Gently lower the sufferer into bath.

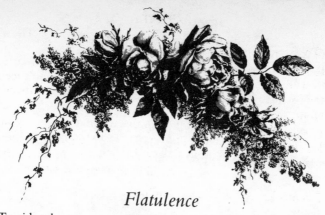

Flatulence

To rid, take a teaspoon bicarbonate of soda in a glass of hot water. Peppermint water will also relieve.

Gargles

These are in the main used to combat sore throats. If only slight, they can be used cold, should it be severe the gargle should be warm. When used to combat a highly infectious or serious infection the gargle should be as hot as possible.

Borax gargle – Mix a pinch of borax and one of salt to half a glass of cold water, stir till dissolved, then use as gargle. It is a good plan to use this each morning as this will strengthen the muscles and cords of the throat.

Chlorate of potash gargle – Add two ounces chlorate of potash to a glass of cold water. Only a little of the chlorate will dissolve, after each gargle top the glass up with more cold water, continue doing this until all is dissolved, keep glass covered.

Gargle for thrush – One part of glycerine to eight of warm water.

Gargle to burst abscess in the throat – One tablespoon washed pearl barley and one of whole linseed. Place in lidded pan add one pint of water, simmer until reduced to half. Use gargle as hot and frequently as possible. Once the abscess has burst use the following:

Healing Gargle – Add two drams tincture of myrrh to a cupful of barley water. Use warm.

Glands (Enlarged)

Paint swelling with tincture of iodine to reduce, give cod liver oil to nourish.

Gout

To relieve pain. Citrate of lithium five to ten grains in a glass of water each morning will prevent the accumulation of the poison. Hot fomentations will give relief.

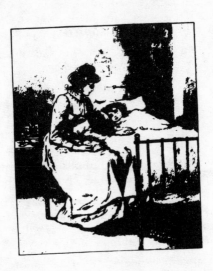

Gravel

Small sand pieces that collect in the kidneys or bladder. This is mainly caused by over indulgence of rich food and drink, or a sluggish liver. Things to avoid if suffering this complaint: sweets, red meat, wine, liquors and malt. The diet should be chicken, mutton, fish, green vegetables and onions. Plenty of barley water as this is of special value.

Gumboils

The mouth should be rinsed with warm Condy's fluid and water.

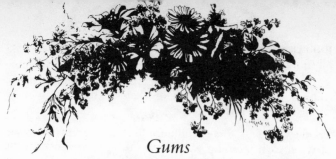

Gums

To harden gums that have receded and loosened teeth in so doing, mix full teaspoon of bicarbonate of soda and just a pinch of alum in a quarter tumbler of water. Wash teeth by holding mixture as long as possible in the mouth, repeat three times daily, as the gums harden so the mixture should be slowly weakened.

Haemorrhoids (Piles)

Find the plant mandrake, peel away its outer layer, crush that which is left to a pulp, mix with lard to ointment consistency, this should then be smoothed onto piles.

Hair

(Loss)

Take burdock roots and stew, strain off the water, drink wineglass full each morning for nine days, leave for nine days and repeat. Continue this treatment for three months. A very effective cure (see also Eczema).

Rub into scalp gas water. Gas water is the water through which coal gas is passed during purification and can be obtained for nothing from the gas works.

(Baldness)

To rectify take of the 'Miracle Brew'. This concoction is listed under Ageing which it also allays.

(Greying – to prevent)

Mix $\frac{1}{16}$th of an ounce of iron sulphate with 9oz red wine. Comb this concoction through hair.

Hands (Chapped and Rough)

Rub with a mixture of mutton fat and caster sugar.

Gather together a bunch of chickweed (it grows in most gardens). Boil in an old saucepan, the water should then be strained into bottles. Rough or chapped hands should be washed only in this liquid.

Harvest Bugs

Bites should be bathed with a solution of warm water with a pinch of bicarbonate of soda added. Once bathed apply sulphur ointment.

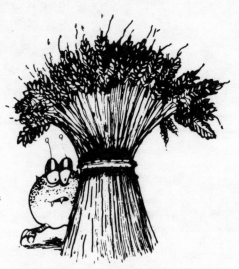

Hay Fever

One tablespoon of lime water *not* lime juice or cordial. The lime water to be taken in a wineglass of milk, three times daily. Preferably start treatment prior to the time of year hay fever usually attacks patient.

To relieve mix a teaspoon of Friar's Balsam to one pint of boiling water, inhale vapour. Boil half pint of milk, to this add glass of sherry, strain, then add sugar to taste, take prior to bedtime.

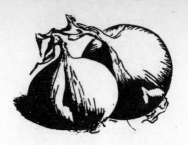

Headache

Rub forehead with a cut onion.

Take a white linen cloth, soak it in vinegar and place on forehead. When dry soak again in vinegar and replace, continue until headache is gone.

Sickly headaches are usually due to indigestion. A little soda water will give relief.

Health

For good health eat raw onion every day. Also boiled nettles and dandelions.

To ensure good health, chop up an onion with a handful of parsley, boil it in rough cider and sweeten with honey. Boil up this liquid, cool and bottle, take two teaspoonsful every night.

Heart (Palpitations)

Indigestion and flatulence are usually the cause. To relieve: half teaspoon of bicarbonate of soda mixed with glass of hot water. Things to avoid: tea, coffee, alcohol and tobacco.

Heartburn

To rid mix half teaspoon of bicarbonate of soda in small glass of peppermint, after which take a glass of hot water.

Heatlumps (or Bee Stings)

Dab with vinegar for relief.

Hypertension

Pick the tender tips of stinging nettles, steep and stew them slowly, strain and bottle the juice. Take one wineglassful every day.

Impetigo

Dust scabs with flowers of sulphur. They will then dry up and drop off.

Indigestion

Causes: irregular times of eating, gulping food and drinking while eating. To cure: ensure meals are regular, only drink once meal is finished. Eat slowly and be sure all food is chewed well before swallowing. Never eat food known to disagree.

Take a handful of rice, steep overnight in teapot. Take a wineglassful every morning. Also good for kidneys.

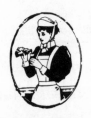

Itch

To treat wash thoroughly using carbolic soap, water as hot as patient can tolerate. Sulphur ointment should be applied at night, take hot bath in morning to remove, repeat till cleared. It is not advisable for others to use towels or flannels of patient.

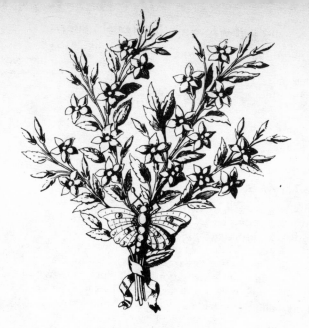

Itch (or Thrush)

Take two Phenogen each night.

Jaundice

Signs: sleepiness, yellowing of eyeballs and highly coloured urine. The diet: milk and broth. Even though with this condition the bowels should be kept free, violent purging is not advised. Simple to prepare remedy: Take one ounce each of senna, camomile flowers, ground ginger and powdered julep, pour boiling water onto ingredients and stir. Take half spoon of mixture twice daily in tea. Ensure complete recovery before getting about or complications might ensue.

Joints (Sprains and Bruises)

Thoroughly soak bandage in *malt* vinegar, apply to the affected part, keep bandages well soaked in the vinegar until relief is obtained. This usually takes only a very short time.

Dissolve camphor in half pint of olive oil, rub this liniment into the affected area.

(Weak and Twisted Legs in Babies and Youngsters)

Gather as many snails as can be found, put into muslin bag, collect the slime that drips through muslin and rub into legs. Continue this treatment every day until legs are normal. (Snails should of course be crushed, care taken to remove all shell.)

Kidneys

(Inflammation)

Cold, damp, scarlet fever, pregnancy can be attributed to cause this complaint. Symptoms are fever, aching loins, headache, vomiting, puffiness of the eyelids, the face becoming pale and swollen. Treatment: the patient should take to their bed, it should be ensured that the temperature of the room is constant, fomentations will reduce pain in loins. The diet should be milk alone, or with soda water. No meat, fish or eggs should be taken. Meat diet should only gradually be returned to in convalescence.

(Stones)

To relieve and dissolve kidney stones (Parsley Breakstone). Gather and dry parsley, infuse in water and drink as required.

Knee (Swollen)

Taking a shovelful of cow dung, heat on the fire until hot, throw into a clean linen cloth and bind around swelling. Continue the treatment daily until swelling subsides. Smelly but effective.

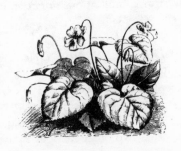

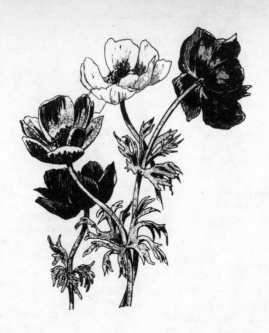

Laxative

Ripe elderberries.

Liver Complaints

Boil up roots of dandelion, take juice whenever feeling liverish.

Remedy, take 1oz of freshly dug dandelion root. Simmer in 1 pint of water till quantity halves, add ½oz compound tincture of horseradish. Use occasionally.

Lumbago

To relieve this condition, wring out a flannel dipped in scalding water, sprinkle with spirits of turpentine and apply to the affected parts. It is also effective to apply belladonna plaster.

Place lump of sugar in a saucer containing oil of juniper, allow the sugar to absorb all the oil it can then eat it slowly. This can be repeated two or three times a day.

Measles

A good handful of marigold flowers boiled in a pint of milk. Strain and drink a cupful at a time.

Isolate the patient. It is wise to be cautious and take care with this infection because of the possible after effects. Ten to eleven days after infection the child develops a fever, loses its appetite, is sleepy and out of sorts; sometimes starts with vomiting and a chill or there may be convulsions. The eyes become reddened and watery. There is a discharge from the nose and a cough. The rash first appears on the face, forehead and behind the ears. It consists of dark red spots that are raised, in patches that run together. The child should be put to bed in a warm well ventilated room, while the eyes are watering the room should be shaded. The cough is the most troublesome symptom, and lest care is taken could develop into bronchitis. Two or three drops of ipecacuanha wine* every four hours will relieve this. The diet should consist mainly of milk while the fever lasts. If the temperature is high and the child restless, the body can be sponged to cool, with tepid water. Particular attention should be given to the patient's eyes, these should be bathed with weak solution of boric acid. A bad cough and difficulty in breathing are bad signs and require specialist treatment. Discharge from the ear should be treated by gently syringing the ear with tepid Condy's fluid, well diluted. The child can leave his sickroom three days after fever is gone, but should not mix with other children for a further three weeks.

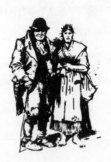

Melancholy

To cure and ensure that sufferer has a happier disposition ensure that plenty of cabbage with honey and salt added is a regular part of diet.

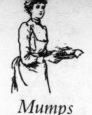

Mumps

Mumps is a very infectious disease, the gland situated below the ear becomes enlarged and inflamed. It occurs mostly in children, who catch it from one another. Two or three weeks after becoming infected the child will complain of feeling ill, or the first sign may be swelling under the ear and pain. There will be stiffness of the jaw and difficulty in eating, inflammation of the throat and tonsils may also occur. About two days after infection is first apparent the other side becomes swollen and painful. The complaint lasts from four to six days, it then starts to get better, normally eight days from the first symptoms the child is all right again. During the illness the bowels should be kept free. The diet should be fluid. The mouth should be washed out with weak Condy's fluid. The patient is infectious for three weeks from onset.

Muscles (Wasted)

Collect as many snails as you can find, put them in a clean container and crush. Collect the frothy green slime that comes from them (minus shell). Massage this frothy substance into the wasted flesh and muscle twice a day.

Nervousness

The best treatment for this disorder is early rising, plenty of exercise preferably out in the fresh air, cheerful company and constant effort to induce confidence. Late meals are not advisable; overstudying and excitement should be avoided.

Night Sweats

Dry patient and remove wet garments, also sheets if dampened. Sponging with lukewarm vinegar and water will help lessen perspiration. A slight dusting of talcum powder is also helpful. In children if these sweats occur in the head it may be a prelude to rickets.

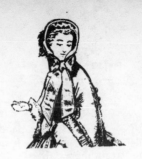

Obesity

Take regular exercise and eat in moderation. Things to partake of sparingly: potatoes, pastry, milk pudding, jams, sugar, fat and bread. Beer and sweet wines are harmful. The diet should consist of lean meat, fish, green vegetables and fruit. Clear soup is preferable to thick, and toast to ordinary bakers bread. For drink use unsweetened fruit, especially lemon or apple juice, and tea with lemon instead of milk or sugar. For general beverage Vichy water is good. A pint of hot water a quarter of an hour before food will, in some cases, reduce weight.

Peppermint Infusion

Steep 6 drams peppermint in 1 pint of boiling water for 15 minutes and then strain. Useful for flatulence, colic, gripe and many other stomach disorders.

Piles

Constipation or the constant taking of strong purgatives, especially those containing aloes, are common causes of piles, as is also chill from sitting on damp surfaces. Treatment consists of avoiding constipation and taking a proper amount of exercise, also care so far as diet is concerned. This should contain liberal allowance of fruit, green vegetables and butter. If the piles bleed they should be treated with witch hazel applied on cotton wool. Once bleeding has ceased an ointment containing the herb pilewort or better known as the lesser celandine, is the best to use.

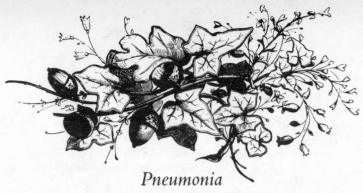

Pneumonia

Wrap top half of patient's body in thermogen wool.

Put boiling water on linseed meal, making a hot paste, put this onto a piece of linen, after which camphorated oil should be sprayed, enough linen should be treated to cover the chest and back.

Poisons (Emetics)

Corrosive poisons. These produce intense agony with swelling of the mouth and throat.
Irritant poisons. The symptoms produced by these are sickness, purging and abdominal pains.
Narcotic poisons. There is no pain, symptoms: giddiness, loss of sight, stupor and sleep and sometimes convulsions.
Narcotic irritants. Symptoms: vomiting and purging of the irritants.

When any poison has been taken it is of the greatest importance that treatment should be given without delay. The first things to do is empty the stomach by means of an emetic (but only if the lips and mouth are not burnt). Do not give emetic for burning poisons such as vitriol, spirits of salt, nitric acid, strong ammonia, caustic soda, carbolic acid, creosote. Then give the right antidote to neutralise the poison which remains in the system. First ensure the patient lies still, apply hot water bottles, give stimulant such as strong coffee or brandy if there are signs of collapse.

For acid poisoning generally, a neutralising antidote quickly at hand in most households is baking powder or bicarbonate of soda, either of which should be given immediately in milk, or in water if milk is not to hand.

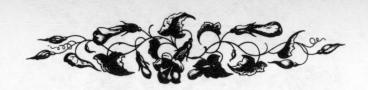

Acetic Acid Chalk and water or white of egg.

Aconite, Monkshood or Blue Rocket Emetic castor oil. Apply hot bottles to feet, give strong coffee.

Alcohol Give emetic, cold water to head and strong ammonia to nose.

Alkalis (Potash, Soda, Ammonia and the like) give drinks containing vinegar or lemonade, lemon juice or olive oil.

Arsenic Emetic; and whites of eggs and milk in large quantities.

Bitter Almond Emetic followed by lots of hot water. Pour cold water on head and face, keep patient warm.

Carbolic Acid Flour and water, or glutinous drinks, such as barley water, whites of egg and milk.

Chloral An emetic and an enema of a pint of strong hot coffee. Wrap in hot blankets; rub and apply hot bottle.

Chloroform An emetic of soda with water. Do everything possible to keep patient from sleeping.

Coal Gas Remove into fresh air, cold water to the head and artificial respiration.

Copper An emetic followed by hot water and barley and water or arrowroot and water.

Deadly Nightshade Emetic, water and big drinks of stewed tea, then strong coffee.

Fish Poisoning Emetic, warm water, castor oil and stimulants.

Foxglove Emetic followed by castor oil and strong tea.

Fungi Emetic, followed by castor oil.

Hemlock Emetic, castor oil or Epsom salts.

Laburnum Mustard and water followed by warm water.

Lead Emetic, then two teaspoons of epsom or glauber salts every two hours, until the bowels are moved. Then give salts in smaller doses.

Morphia (Opium, Laudanum) Emetic. If the patient is able to swallow a solution of permanganate of potash, a pinch to a pint of water should be given and repeated. Condy's fluid in water has the same effect as an antidote. The patient must be kept awake and mobile. As he becomes more sensible give hot strong tea or coffee.

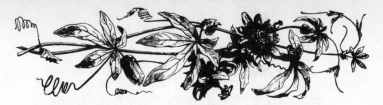

Mushrooms Emetic, and a big dose of castor oil or salts.

Nicotine Emetic, douche head and face with cold water, and give tea, coffee, or alcohol.

Nitric Acid Force down some chalk and water and afterwards large draughts of plain barley water.

Oxalic Acid (Acid of Sugar) Magnesia or chalk and water, then castor oil.

Paraffin Oil Emetic, tea and coffee.

Phosphorus Emetic, a weak solution of Condy's fluid should be given. Epsom salts. Castor oil should not be given as this causes the poison to act more quickly.

Prussic Acid Emetic. Cold water in a jug should be poured over head and chest. Give teaspoon of sal volatile in water. The speed with which this poison acts renders treatment difficult. The patient becomes insensible at once, and nothing can be done but remove them to the open air and pour cold water over their head and chest.

Ptomaine Emetics followed by purgatives. Brandy if needed.

Salts of Lemon Encourage vomiting by tickling back of throat. Water should not be given as this would dissolve the acid and it would act more quickly. Whiting, the thickness of gruel should be given.

Spanish Fly Blistering fluids – Emetic, warm water, no oils should be given as this hastens the action of the poison.

Spirits of Salt Chalk mixed with water; give barley water.

Strychnine Emetics and strong tea, the tannin acts as an antidote.

Sugar of Lead Emetic, and a big dose of Epsom salts, egg and milk.

Sulphuric Acid (Oil of Vitriol) Chalk mixed with water; give barley water or linseed tea.

Turpentine Emetic, Epsom salts, egg and milk, barley water.

Yew Twigs and Fruit Emetic, Epsom salts or castor oil.

(Editor's note: in cases of poisoning, a doctor should always be consulted first. As with all Grandmother's Cures, these treatments are not recommended.)

Poultice

(Bread)

After removing crusts place slice of bread in bowl then pour boiling water onto it. Cover bowl with plate and leave for a while, preferably in front of fire. Strain pulped bread with fork and spread where needed.

(Dry Poultice)

Make cloth bag size needed, fill with bran, place in oven leave till hotted thoroughly, then apply where needed.

(Jacket)

Used for cases of pneumonia. Two large linseed poultices should be prepared. Apply one to chest the other to the back. They must be large enough to meet on shoulders and under arms.

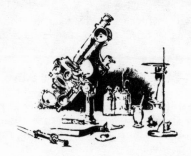

Quinsy

To cure: take a slice of rusty bacon i.e. bacon that has been smoked, tie this around the throat when retiring to bed, rusty side (rind) towards the skin. By morning the quinsy should have broken and the throat become easier.

Take one warm fresh cowpat, wrap in muslin and bind around throat. Unpleasant but very effective.

Bake a potato in its jacket, drop into sock and put hot around patients neck.

Take one dessertspoonful of goose grease.

Heat a quantity of salt, when hot put into an old sock or stocking and tie around throat, this should break the quinsy.

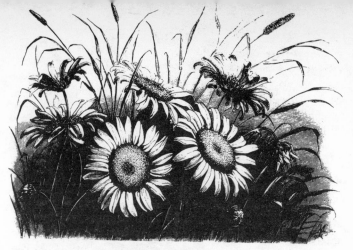

Relaxed Throat

Causes: excessive use of voice, over indulgence in tobacco and alcohol. Symptoms: sore throat and the person continually attempts to clear throat. The glands in the neck may enlarge. Treatment: rest the voice, moderation in smoking and drinking. The throat should be gargled night and morning with lukewarm Condy's fluid. Parrish's food – a teaspoon three times a day – will act as a tonic.

Rheumatics

To cure: swallow a small frog – for effective cure the frog must be alive when eaten.

To stop pain: sting the affected part with nettles. The sting of the nettles will be painful for about two minutes, then the pain will go, leaving only a tingle which is not unpleasant.

Drink strained water of boiled stinging nettles. Or carry a raw potato in pocket.

Rheumatism

Treatment: mix equal parts of oil of wintergreen and olive oil, rub this into affected joints and muscles. Medicine: a tried and excellent remedy is a concoction made up of 1oz sulphur; 1oz cream of tartar; 1oz rhubarb; 1 dram gum guiacum; 16oz honey. Take a teaspoon or more morning and night.

(Muscular)

Treatment: Rest and applications of hot flannels. The part may be covered with a cloth and a hot iron run over. Massage, Turkish baths give relief. Great care must be taken that the patient does not catch cold after bath, as this will make condition worsen. Should the pain become troublesome, give ten grains of salicylate of soda to relieve.

Ringworm

This is a very contagious infection. Wash the affected area with iodine or antispetic lotion after removing hair around the sore. Ensure cleanliness of area, and application of precipitate ointment at intervals.

Crush the leaves of the house leek and apply, also good for corns. Must be used for a few days to ensure cure.

Stockholm tar. Warm slightly and spread over infection.

Scalds

Rub goose grease onto affected area.

Sciatica

Bathe affected area with hot water. Mix 2oz camphorated oil, 1oz ammonia in ¼ pint of turpentine. After thorough shaking use to rub onto affected parts.

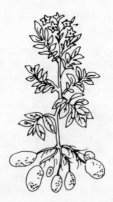

Shingles

This condition is usually the result of a chill. The most likely places it occurs are around the mouth corners, on the neck, arm, chest and waist. Symptoms: it erupts as small blisters on an inflamed base. The eruptions are painful tingles and smart, they always follow the course of a nerve. If the blisters break and become infected, or the patient irritates them by scratching, alarming sores may develop. Treatment: zinc ointment or powdered starch and zinc oxide should be applied. If the blisters break and leave a raw area, it should be dusted at once or the ointment applied. A raw surface should never be allowed to be exposed to air, neither should clothes be allowed to touch it. A ten grain dose of antipyrin will relieve pain and smarting.

Scrape the koom, a green fungi (verdigris) from a church bell, mix with Vaseline, apply to infection.

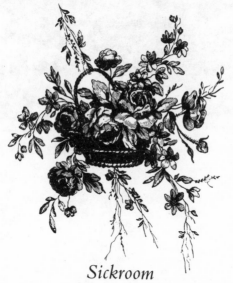

Sickroom

To purify air in a sickroom, burn sulphur candles.

Sinus Trouble

Place a small quantity of camphorated oil up each nostril, this will stop irritation and release mucus obstructing sinus. Continue treatment until pain and discomfort cease.

Sleeplessness

Place hops in pillow.

Should indigestion be the cause then diet should be checked. An overactive mind can be calmed by taking a walk prior to retiring. A biscuit and glass of hot milk or home-made lemonade is an excellent sleeping draught. A tepid bath and hot water bottle to feet are in most cases sufficient to induce sleep. Drugs of any form are dangerous, sleeping draughts are not advised.

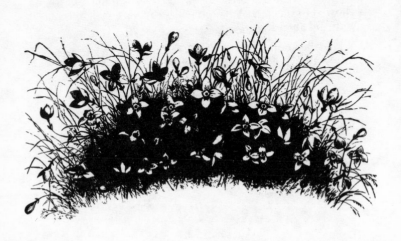

Smallpox

Soak gauze squares in camphor oil, place in brassière or vest.

Sores

(Bleeding)

Scatter white pepper on minor sores or wounds, this will stop bleeding and aid recovery.

(Open)

Scorch piece of white linen in front of coal fire and bind. Repeat twice daily. This is also good for ulcerated wounds.

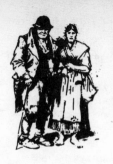

Sprained Ankle

Wash ankle frequently with salted cold water. Dry lightly but thoroughly. Keep the ankle as cool as possible to prevent inflammation, try to keep feet elevated. Massage gently with liniment, repeat treatment at intervals.

Starch Bath

Two tablespoons of starch dissolved and added to bath acts as an excellent tonic for the skin.

Stings

(Bee)

Dab with vinegar.

Cut onion in half, rub on sting. This will stop the swelling and the pain. (Bee and wasp.)

(Nettle)

To bring relief spit on dockleaf and place or rub over affected area.

Rub with rosemary, sage or mint leaves.

(Rash)

To rid, boil some young nettle tops and drink the juice.

(Wasp)

To relieve wasp sting in the mouth suck raw onion.

Stings and Bites

Prevent by sponging body after morning bath with solution comprising of dessertspoonful of Epsom salts in three pints of water. Just before going out put a drop of the oil of citronella onto old handkerchief, to pin on hat or coat when insects are about. To treat rub onto the bitten parts either camphorated oil or a solution of one part carbolic acid in ten parts of oil. Other simple remedies that may be carried in the pocket or handbag, are a piece of soda or carbonate of ammonia finely crushed. If a bite becomes inflamed it should be bathed with a solution of warm boracic acid lotion. Starch powder is effective.

(Wasp and Bee stings)

The sting may protrude, if so it should be removed immediately. If it does not the best way to get it above the skin is to place over the spot a hollow key or something of that nature, and press it to force the sting sufficiently out so enabling it to be removed using tweezers. Then apply either iodine, sal volatile, vinegar, juice of an onion or soda solution. Not only will the pain be reduced, the swelling will also.

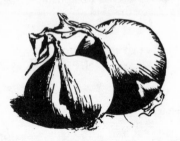

Stomach Ache (or Disorder)

Drink a cupful of hot wormwood tea made by simmering wormwood for two hours and decanting off.

(Inflammation of)

Treatment: the bowels should be emptied by means of an enema. No food should be taken in solid form. The only food to be given should be liquid form, such as gruel, milk and water, or tea made with milk. Should the patient require a drink iced water should be given. Fomentations should be applied to stomach.

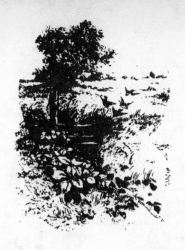

Stuttering

To cure, brew a strong solution of ivy leaves and with a cloth soaked in the infusion, bathe the outside of the throat.

Styes and Sore Eyes

Bathe with bag containing soaked tea leaves.

Teething Problems (Baby)

To allay: gather young elderberry shoots, cut them into small pieces and then thread them as a necklace. Tie around the baby's neck.

Tension

To relieve: take a brown paper bag, breathe into bag, ensure you breathe back that air you breathed out. Do this for about thirty seconds and tension will be relieved.

Thorn (Embedded)

To remove: scald a piece of white bread, squeeze out surplus water, press the bread onto embedded thorn, bandage and leave. The thorn will be drawn out.

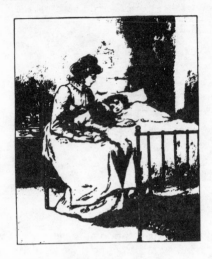

Throat (Sore)

Take large onion, slice into layers approximately quarter inch thick. Cover bottom layer with as much demerara sugar as will go, after placing in saucer. Replace next layer, and repeat with sugar. Do this until onion is as whole again. Leave overnight, or all day, as the case may be. After this time the saucer will contain a brown syrup. Take two spoonsful in the morning and the same at night.

A woollen sock after being worn, put around the throat when going to bed will cure a sore throat.

Put flowers of sulphur into a paper funnel, insert small end into patient's mouth. Blow into other and thus ensuring fumes from the flowers of sulphur penetrate and cure sore throat.

Put rasher of bacon around throat and leave overnight.

Simmer gently a handful of linseed in 2 pints of hot water until mass becomes jellified. Add 1 ounce of black liquorice stick, 2 ounces of liquorice root and juice of 2 lemons and simmer further. Keep hot on hob and drink half a teacup three or four times a day.

Tongue

To examine for symptoms: brown or black tongue indicates blood poisoning; dry tongue – feverishness; strawberry coloured – scarlet fever; white coated tongue – disordered stomach; yellow coated – disordered liver. It is a good sign when the tongue clears gradually from the edge.

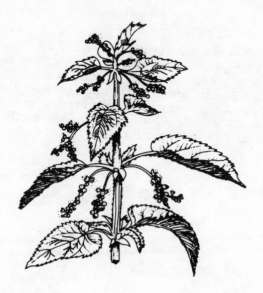

Tonic

Empty a bottle of good strong beer into a saucepan, add a knob of butter, a pinch of ground ginger and sugar to taste. Heat this gently but thoroughly and drink when going to bed.

(Orange)

Steep in 1 pint of boiling water 1oz of orange peel, 1oz of camomile flowers and a few cloves.

(Children's Bitter Herbs)

Collect bunch of stinging nettles, cut off at six inch lengths, stand in jug, pour boiling water over them. When water has cooled bottle liquid and give spoonsful to children as required.

Toothache

Press a cayenne onto tooth.

Cut a six inch square of brown paper, sprinkle on a few drops of vinegar and some pepper, place on jaw and hold in place with a woollen scarf around the head. The pain will soon be eased.

Place a clove in mouth, as near to offending tooth as possible.

Bind a slice of horseradish onto the wrist on the side opposite to the offending tooth.

Soak soft brown paper in warm malt vinegar and hold on cheek where tooth aches. In severe cases dissolve as much camphor as possible in a dram of nitre, to which add two spots of ammonia. Insert a tiny fragment of cotton wool into the split end of a match stalk, dip into the mixture then press on to centre of hollow of tooth affected. Patient should be warned to spit out and not to swallow.

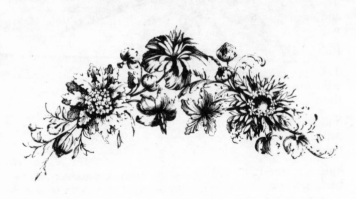

Tuberculosis

Collect and dry rosemary; once dried it should be smoked. This will bring relief and eventually rid patient of ailment.

Vomiting

An effective means of stopping vomiting is to drink water as hot as can be taken, or cold water if the cause is bilious nausea.

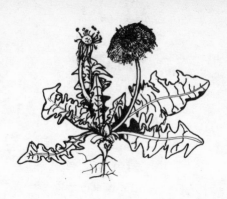

Warts

To rid, mix together ½oz acetic acid and ½oz tincture steel and apply by rubbing well on warts twice daily. The wart will shrink and fall off within a few days.

Rub with radish or sloe berries.

Take one horsehair (can be found on the fence around fields where horses are kept), wind tightly around wart. Within a short time the wart will turn black and drop off.

Squeeze the white milky substance out of the stem of the dandelion on to the warts, or rub spittle on them first thing in the morning.

Take a piece of raw beef, rub over warts, bury the beef. As beef rots away so will offending warts.

Wet and soften the head of a red top match, do this with spittle. Rub on and around wart, repeat every night for a week, at the end of this time the wart will fall off.

Take a lump of common household soda, once daily wet with spittle and rub over warts. Continue treatment (take care to use the same piece of soda all the time) until warts disappear.

Brush warts with an elderberry flower, throw the flower over the left shoulder, under no circumstances look to where it has fallen.

Take some blood from a freshly killed pig and rub onto warts. The warts will then gradually disappear.

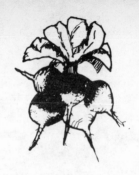

Whitlows

To cure: take the leaf of the wild marsh mallow, wash and wrap onto whitlow.

Take a lily of the valley leaf which has been soaked in brandy, wrap around whitlow. This should effect a cure within two days.

Take the leaves of the common mallow plant, steep several in boiling water for two to three minutes. Use as poultice on the affected part keeping it in place with a bandage. Repeat treatment until swelling subsides.

Whooping Cough

Its beginning is likened to that of a cold on the chest, the coughing increases and comes in spasms. It is also accompanied by slight fever, after onset. Treatment: Isolation and lots of fresh air. The greatest care must be taken with the child convalescent, rub chest with warm camphorated oil, and hang around the neck menthol crystals sewn in muslin bag, this will ease child's breathing. *Do not apply poultices.*

Ensure patient gets plenty of fresh sea air.

Take a *new laid* egg and cover it with vinegar for twenty-four hours. The shell dissolves in vinegar. To this liquid add honey, the mixture must then be stirred with red hot poker. A few spoonsful will cure even the worst cough.

Catch and kill two mice, prepare as for rabbit and bake. Give to patient to eat. This should cure whooping cough within two days.

Tie a moleskin around the neck to bring relief.

Cut a hair from a donkey's back where the cross appears, and place in a silken purse to be hung around the sufferer's neck.

The sufferer should be taken if possible for a walk around sheep pens, or hang a piece of tarred rope in pram or cot (for a child) or burn a coal tar lamp or candle in the room.

Slice a turnip and a swede. Put into large bowl first a layer of turnip, cover this with a layer of sugar; place a layer of swede onto this, sprinkle a further layer of sugar. Continue doing this until swede and turnip are used up, leave for twenty-four hours. This produces a liquid which should be given a few spoonsful at a time to the patient until relief is obtained.

Encourage patient to inhale fumes from hot tar.

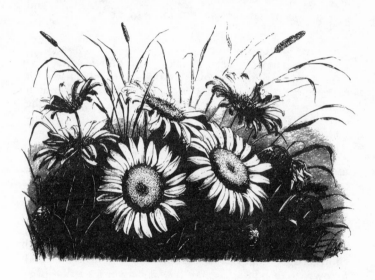

Wind in Stomach

To treat young children boil with their food a piece of ginger, or a few caraway seeds. Older children should be given a few drops of strong peppermint water on a piece of sugar. For adults one teaspoon of ordinary bicarbonate of soda in hot water, this can be taken alone or with peppermint water.

To relieve a baby suffering with wind, the child should be given cinder tea. To make is simple: take one red hot cinder, place in a cupful of boiling water, allow to cool, strain and give teaspoon when needed.

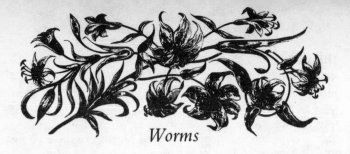

Worms

(Round)

Symptoms: Abdominal pains may be present, capricious appetite, itching at the nose. As a rule, however, the worms give rise to no symptoms. The first one knows of their presence, is when seen in the motions or when they are vomited.

Treatment 1: The person should take a dose of salts and abstain from food for a few hours. After the bowels have been moved, administer a worm cake, this can be obtained from the chemist. Once this has had time to work, a dose of liquorice or Gregory powder will expel the parasite. The treatment should be repeated as the worms take a lot of killing.

Treatment 2: To 1 teaspoon of common salt add 1 pint of warm water. Inject night and morning, allow to remain in bowels as long as possible. Give patient plenty of fresh fruit.

(Tape)

Take two teaspoons of powdered kamala first thing on rising. If the bowels are not moved in approximately two hours then a further spoonful of kamala should be taken. This should be followed two hours later by taking between a half to one ounce of castor oil. This is a certain cure for tapeworm and causes no sickness.

(Thread)

These infest the lower part of the bowels and their presence is recognisable by the fact they give rise to heat and irritation around the anus. Treatment is simple. Ensure these parts are kept very clean and washed in warm water and soap. The diet should be regulated and sweets avoided. A dose of castor oil or magnesia should be given. After this has acted, a solution of salt water (1 teaspoon of salt to 12 teaspoons of tepid water) should be injected into the bowels with a syringe.

Wounds

(Bleeding)

Sprinkle with pepper, does not sting – aids healing and stops bleeding.

Take one thick black cobweb and lay on the cut, bind up. This will staunch the blood flow and heal up wound without any festering.

(Comfrey Poultice)

Scald comfrey with boiling water, squeeze and apply to wound.

(Cuts)

Make a batch of curd tarts: Cream together ¼lb butter, 3oz sugar, add ½lb curd, 3oz currants, 1 tablespoon flour and 2 beaten eggs. Flavour with nutmeg, mix well and bake in a quick oven. These should be left to go mouldy and the mould rubbed upon open cuts whether minor or serious. Very effective.

Take mould off the top of jam and rub on wound before bandaging.

(Poisonous Bite)

Cut the affected part with a sharp knife immediately, squeeze or suck out poison.

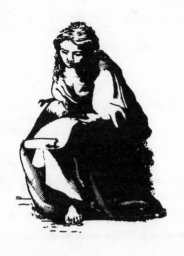

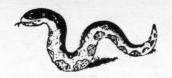

(Septic)

This should not occur if a fresh wound is cleaned immediately on occurrence and sterilised with a solution of pure carbolic acid crystals. Should a wound turn septic however, for slight cases, use a linseed meal poultice by mixing the meal in a teacup with boiling water and apply as hot as possible, changing twice daily. For more severe cases, bathe first with an infusion of leaves of marsh mallow, wormwood and mugwort – using as hot as possible, then poultice frequently with slippery elm.

Gather a handful of plantain leaves and chickweed. Wash and place on wound, bind over with clean cloth.

To draw out pus use soap and sugar poultice. Mix soap and sugar together into a paste. Take a piece of brown paper, cut a hole large enough to allow head of infected wound to protrude, spread paste onto the brown paper. Place over sore, this will draw out pus and is very effective.

Cut a piece of pink boracic lint, prepare a mixture of washing soap and sugar, spread a film of this onto the lint. Boil a kettle and holding the lint with scissors or tweezers allow the steam from the kettle spout to melt the soap/sugar mixture a little, ensuring the mixture is quite hot. Place immediately onto the septic wound, strap down and leave for about eight hours depending upon progress of the wound, repeat two or three times more. If necessary in some cases, sterilise a needle by holding over a flame and pierce the wound to allow the poison to escape.

Put a piece of snakeskin (sloughed off by the snake during spring) on the infection, bind with bandage. Within a day or two the infection will be cured.

Collect fungus from the bottom of a beech tree, mix with Vaseline, use as required.

Make an ointment of leaf lard (can be bought at butcher's) beeswax and burgundy pitch. Render lard slowly over gentle heat to avoid burning. The clear fat should then be poured into a pan to which should be added beeswax and burgundy pitch. When evenly mixed, mixture should be poured into jar to solidify, then it will be ready for use.

Wrinkles

To prevent: use a gentle massage of glycerine and honey, apply a small quantity to the face on retiring. Wash in warm rainwater next morning using unscented white curd soap.

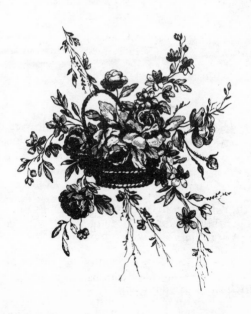

PART TWO

MOTHER NATURE'S MEDICINE CABINET

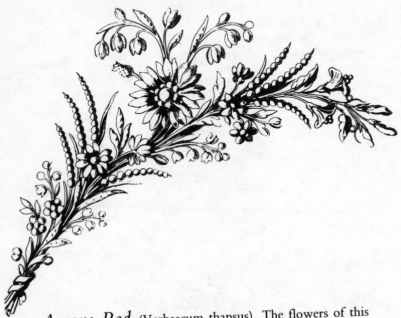

Aarons Rod (Verbascum thapsus). The flowers of this plant much used by herbalists to ease coughs and chills, after drying they would later infuse to a medicine.

Agrimony (Agrimonia eupatoria). Recommended should one feel liverish, good for the eyesight, also relieves amnesia. An infusion of the leaves make a refreshing alternative to tea.

Alexanders (Smyrnium olusatrum). The black seeds of this have long been used by herbalists as a cure for flatulence and for warming the stomach, also as a cure against snake bites.

Angelica, Wild (Angelica sylvestris). The roots and seeds of this plant have been used and acclaimed for their wondrous medicinal properties by herbalists for many years.

Apple, Crab (Malus sylvestris). Apothecaries used the juices acquired by fermenting the fruits of this tree to cure scalds and sprains.

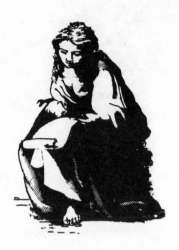

Barberry (Berberis vulgaris). People of yesteryear did not suffer the common cold as we do today for they were aware of the abundant amount of vitamin C contained within the berries of this shrub, and made jams and jellies from them. Also said to cure liver and stomach complaints.

Bartsia, Red (Odontites verna). Used as a cure for tooth-ache.

Bay, Sweet (Laurus nobilis). The leaves of this shrub were used as a cleanser of the inner body. Laxative, also reckoned to cure troublesome coughs.

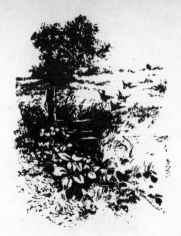

Bilberry (Vaccinium myrtillus). The fruit of this plant contains a high percentage of vitamins C and D, also used as a cure for diarrhoea.

Bistort (Polygonum bistorta). Contains astringent properties, used extensively in early times to arrest internal and external bleeding, also used to treat various infectious diseases.

Bog Bean (Menyanthes trifoliata). Claimed to be a cure for scurvy and a good blood purifier. Used by many herbalists as a general tonic.

Borage (Borago officinalis). Extracts from this plant are used to treat fevers and nervous complaints.

Brooklime (Veronica beccabunga). A plant liking the very damp banks of streams, when steeped produces a drink very good for purging the blood. Herbalists of the 17th Century claimed the plant was a cure for scurvy. It was also said to be like to spices (hot to the mouth) when fried in batter and vinegar, and used to relieve tumours, swelling and inflammations.

Bugle (Ajuga reptans). This plant was said to be a cure for most ailments, no medicine cabinet was complete without the syrup concocted from it contained within. Also recommended highly to combat a hangover. It is a mild narcotic.

Burnet, Great (Sanguisorba officinalis). Plant used by early herbalists to stop bleeding, the root freshly dug and peeled then applied to burns is said to soothe and encourage healing.

Butterbur (Petasites hybridus). The powdered root of this plant was said to cure unsightly blemishes of the skin, also spots.

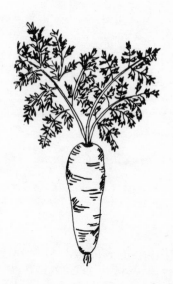

Carrot, Wild (Daucus carota). The juices from this plant were deemed by herbalists in the 17th Century to possess fertility powers. Any woman failing to conceive and seeking their advice would have been instructed to boil the wild carrot in wine and drink of this to help conception.

Celandine, Greater (Chelidonium majus). The sap of this plant was used to burn away warts and corns. As the sap is caustic it should be used with great care.

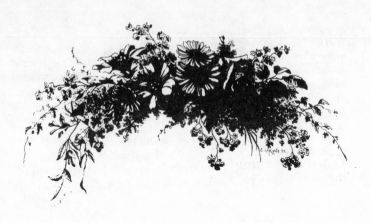

Celandine, Lesser (Ranunculus ficaria). It is claimed by Nicholas Culpeper, a renowned herbalist of the 17th Century, that he cured his daughter of scrofula with the use of this plant. Scrofula is a swelling of the glands of the neck.

Centaury, Common (Centaurium erythraea). So called after the creature, part horse and part man, said to have used the plant to heal a wound. One herbalist claimed it removed freckles and other facial blemishes.

Cherry, Bird (Prunus padus). An infusion of the bark of this tree was prescribed to cure stomach disorders, also as a tonic to ensure freedom from such complaints.

Cherry, Wild (Prunus avium). The medicinal properties of the fruits produced by this tree have long been known, and used in cough mixtures and syrups.

Cicely, Sweet (Myrrhis odorata). The roots boiled and eaten with a sprinkling of vinegar and oil was claimed to stimulate the elderly, the seeds were used as a remedy for rheumatics.

Clover, Red (Trifolium pratense). Herbalists and Romanies were well aware of the relief syrup made up from this plant brought to sufferers of whooping cough, also the medicinal properties of honey collected from any bumble bee nest that happened to be in a hedge or woods near a field containing this plant.

Corn Cromwell (Buglossoides arvensis). An infusion of the seeds of this plant was said to dissolve kidney stones.

Cranberry (Vaccinium oxycoccos). Not thought highly of regarding its medicinal properties, that is lest crossed in love and suffering with a broken heart; it was claimed the cranberry would ease the pain. So suffer no more fair maiden with the pangs of a broken heart, take of the cranberry and the pain will be gone.

Creeping Jenny (Lysimachia nummularia). In the reign of James I, it was believed by many herbalists that this plant contained properties that relieved pain, and had great faith in its healing qualities.

Cuckoo Flower (Cardamine pratensis). This plant, although often used as a substitute for watercress, has not often been used for its medicinal properties because of the superstitions that surround it.

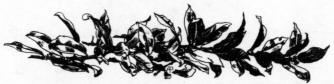

Daffodil (Narcissus pseudonarcissus). The bulb of this abundant plant was used as a purge. To administer, it was ground to a powder and mixed with cereal. This was said to have the ability to dismiss all obstructions.

Daisy (Bellis perennis). A claimed cure for consumption was to boil this plant in asses' milk and take of its infusion.

Daisy, Ox-Eye (Leucanthemum vulgare). This plant was much used for its medical properties. To name but a few: an infusion of this plant was prescribed to combat chest and liver ailments, the juices of the stems were recommended in the treatment of weary and sore eyes.

Dandelion (Taraxacum officinale). An infusion of this plant is said to work wonders, a good cleanser of the liver and purifier of the blood.

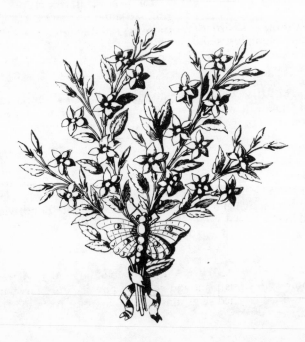

Dock, Curled (Rumex crispus). Used to neutralise the sting of nettles, also as a healant for burns, scalds and blisters.

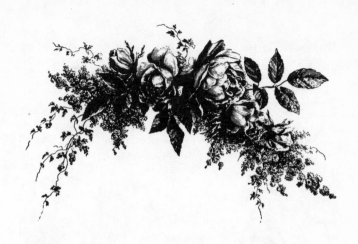

Dodder, Common (Cuscuta epithymum). Liver and kidney complaints and many other diseases were treated by herbalists using a concoction made by boiling the stems of this plant, especially if the host plant was wild thyme. One can only conclude that the blending of these two plants attributed to its high medicinal properties.

Dog Rose (Rosa canina). It was claimed by ancient Greeks that the roots of this plant contained medicinal properties, able to cure anyone that was bitten by a mad dog. Apart from this, because of its high content of vitamin C in the rose hips, another medicinal use the plant has, is as a syrup for growing children.

Dove's-foot Crane's-Bill (Geranium molle). To treat ruptures, dry this plant and crush to powder, mix this with oven-dried crushed slugs; this concoction to be taken in glass of claret.

Elder (Sambucus nigra). The flowers of this shrub were at one time dried and then infused and drunk as tea. This was claimed to prevent and cure the cold. The flowers are very rich in vitamin C.

Elder, Ground (Aegopodium podagraria). Said to be a cure for gout.

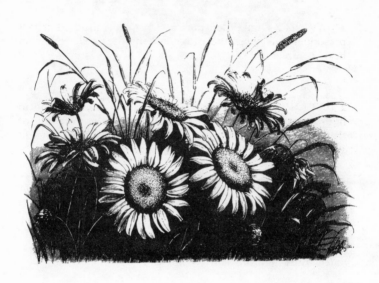

Fever Few (Tanacetum parthenium). A plant held in high esteem for its curative properties. Apart from its known ability to dispel fevers, it was claimed to cure many illnesses suffered by women and was also highly recommended to them prior to and after childbearing.

Fleabane (Pulicaria dysenterica). Though this plant has no known medicinal qualities, it played an important part in the control of diseases because of its pesticide ingredients. To fleas, who must have been one of the main transporters of disease, the fumes from this plant meant certain death.

Figwort, Common (Scrophularia nodosa). Claimed to be a cure by early herbalists for diseases affecting the neck glands, such as scrofula. The leaves were also used to treat all types of skin diseases, gangrene included.

Forget-Me-Not (Myosotis arvensis). Syrup made from any of this group of plants was claimed by herbalists to be a cure for lung ailments, also a good cough cure.

Foxglove (Digitalis purpurea). This plant, although in fact poisonous, produces the drug digitalis used extensively in heart complaints.

Foxglove Tree (Paulownia tomentosa). A tree held in high esteem by the Chinese. It was claimed 'not greying of the hair nor wrinkling of the skin would you suffer' should you take of an infusion of the leaves and fruit of this tree.

Fumitory (Corydalis claviculata). Much renowned for its cure of intestinal diseases.

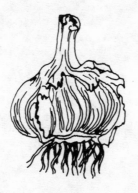

Garlic, Cultivated (Allium ursinum). The juices of this plant have strong antiseptic values, and well documented healing abilities.

Gentian, Autumn (Gentiana amarella). This plant was able to cure the same ailments as field and marsh gentians. It was also used to cure cramp, scrofula and loss of appetite.

Gentian, Field (Gentianella campestris). This plant also cures poisonous bites; it also puts to right stomach disorders, for this the roots need to be powdered.

Gentian, Marsh (Gentiana pneumonanthe). It is said the roots of this plant can be used as an antidote to poisonous bites.

Grass of Parnassus (Parnassia palustris). Herbalists used this plant to correct liver complaints. It was also said that an infusion of the leaves would rid one of kidney stones.

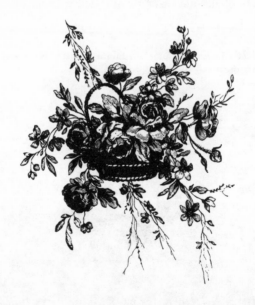

Herb-robert (Geranium robertianum). In the middle ages this plant was used for blood disorders, also to stop bleeding.

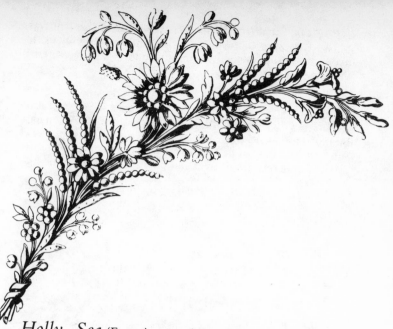

Holly, Sea (Eryngium maritimum). For many years the roots of this plant were gathered from the shores of the east coast of England, and sold as a delicacy. It was claimed by some that these roots were in fact an aphrodisiac and should be regularly eaten by the elderly; thus they would be restored to youthful vitality.

Honeysuckle (Lonicera pericylmenum). A concoction of the flowers would be recommended for those who suffered asthmatic attacks, lung diseases or headaches.

Hop (Humulus lupulus). Should one suffer of tension, it is said 'to place of the hop in that person's pillow this tension shall be eased and restful sleep induced.'

Hound's Tongue (Cynoglossum officinale). Bites from mad dogs were treated by binding the leaf of this plant directly onto such a bite; also used to prevent baldness and in some cases, cure it.

Juniper, Common (Juniperus communis). The berries of this tree were claimed to be an effective antidote against many poisons, a concoction made from them was said to cure the bite of a frenzied dog.

Knapweed, Greater (Centaurea scabiosa). A concoction of this plant was said to relieve and cure those that suffered bruising, to be taken with wine. The plant was also used by apothecaries to treat and cure many other ailments.

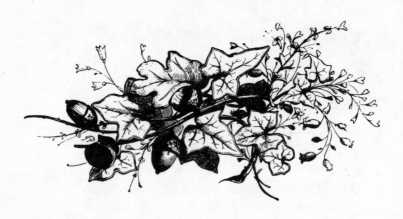

Ladies' Bedstraw (Galium verum). This plant contains medicinal properties that prevent blood clotting. These medicinal abilities have been known to herbalists for many years, and have been used by them to treat bladder and kidney complaints. It is also highly recommended as a relaxant to be added to bathing water.

Ladies' Mantle (Alchemilla vulgaris). Herbalists in bygone days claimed that this plant produced that which was needed to cure many womanly ailments, and that it also had the power to restore sagging breasts to a youthful firmness.

Lily of the Valley (Convallaria majalis). To take of this plant was said to encourage greater capability of the brain; was also reckoned to rejuvenate a mind feeble with age.

Loosestrife, Yellow (Lysimachia vulgaris). Many years ago used as a fly and insect repellent. Its medicinal use as implied by its name, was to remove strife.

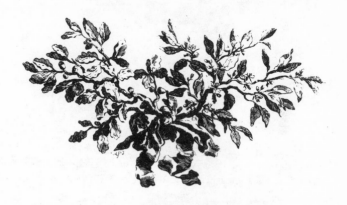

Mallow, Common (Malva sylvestris). Young ladies of bygone days feared not the advances of an ardent lover, for they were aware of the powers of this plant as an anti aphrodisiac. Just a drop of its sap in a glass of water would cool even the most persistant. Also recommended to rid one of a hangover, even the worst such as from a night of orgies and heavy drinking. It is also claimed to be good for stings and its sap was used to make a fine ointment.

Marjoram, Wild (Origanum vulgare). It is claimed the leaves of this plant, powdered, cures many ills.

Mayweed, Scented (Chamomilla recutita). Take of the tea concocted from this plant and it is claimed you should suffer no more sleepless nights, nor the pangs of indigestion.

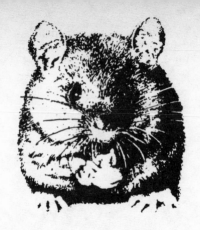

Mayweed, Scentless (Matricaria maritima). A plant used much by herbalists to rectify womanly problems.

Meadow Rue, Common (Thalictrum flavum). This plant contains no known useful medicinal properties, although the leaves and roots make an excellent purgative.

Meadowsweet (Filipendula ulmaria). Used much as an early air freshener, its fragrance much sweeter than that of dank musk. It was also claimed, 'he that taketh of an infusion of this plant banished his aches and pains.' It was also used to break fevers.

Medlar (Mespilus germanica). The fruits of this tree were used by herbalists to cure many things, staunching excessive bleeding, ridding stones from the kidney and curing stomach ailments.

Milkwort, Common (Polygala vulgaris). A concoction made from this plant was recommended to mothers breastfeeding, for it was said to stimulate and increase the flow of milk.

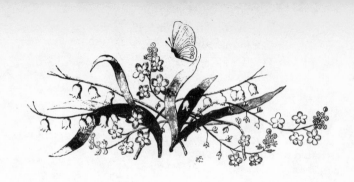

Mint Water (Mentha aquatica).

A lady of yesteryear feeling faint would almost certainly have had a hanky wafted beneath her nose containing this plant, just enough being crushed to release its beneficial fragrance to assist her revival.

Mullein, Dark (Verbascum nigrum).

Even though poisonous to animals if eaten in any quantity, one herbalist claimed that a concoction made from the leaves of this plant eased chest complaints such as coughing and spitting blood.

Mustard, Black (Brassica nigra).

Said to cure a cold by soaking the feet in a hot mustard bath. Also highly recommended as a poultice to relieve chest ailments, or to banish muscular pains.

Mustard, Hedge (Sisymbrium officinale).

A plant which many a person who use their voice to excess (such as singers, politicians and actors) attribute their fine tone of voice. They gargle with an infusion made from this plant.

Mustard, Treacle (Erysimum cheiranthoides).

Recommended by early herbalists as an antidote against poisonous bites and stings. Songs of praise were often sung acclaiming the curing abilities of this plant. It is said the seeds would rid the infant of worms.

Nettle, Stinging (Urtica dioica). Suffer no more the scourge of modern man: hypertension. To rid: take an infusion of this plant, also claimed by many to be capable of curing rheumatism.

Nodding Bur-Marigold (Bidens cernua). It was claimed a concoction obtained by infusion of all this plant was effective treatment for lung diseases.

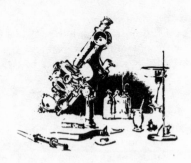

Orache, Common (Atriplex patula). Can be used as a gentle laxative. Because of this quality, even though it is rich in vitamin C, this plant is rarely used.

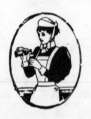

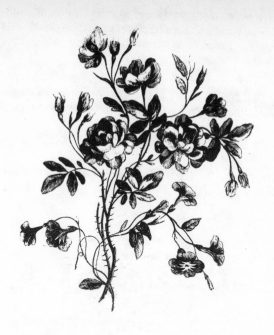

Parsley Piert (Aphanes arvensis). Used by herbalists to right intestinal disorders.

Parsnip, Wild (Pastinaca sativa). An infusion made from the roots of this plant was said to put to right kidney disorders, and rid any obstruction from the intestines.

Pennyroyal (Mentha pulegium). Used to cure many ailments, also to rid households and people of fleas.

Pennywort, Marsh (Hydrocotyle vulgaris). Said to be able to rid the stone from the body.

Perforate St. John's Wart (Hypericum perforatum). This plant was believed to be able to cure all open wounds.

Periwinkle, Lesser (Vinca minor). For the treatment of love strained and waning. Together eat the leaves of this plant to regain the love you once shared and enjoyed.

Pimpernel, Scarlet (Anagallis arvensis). An infusion of this plant when taken is said to bring happiness even to those that are depressed.

Pimpernel, Yellow (Lysimachia nemorum). Used extensively at one time as a painkiller.

Plantain, Buck's Horn (Plantago coronopus). The leaves of this plant were used effectively to treat open sores, and should one have the mishap to be bitten by a mad dog, it was claimed this plant had the ability to protect against infection.

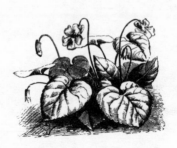

Primrose (Primula vulgaris). Fear not the loss of thy loved one, for should you give them a concoction infused from the flower of the primrose their love shall be yours forever.

Privet, Oval Leaved (Ligustrum ovalifolium). An infusion of the leaves of this shrub was much used at one time as a gargle. It was said to rid one of ulcers of the mouth or throat and reduce swollen glands.

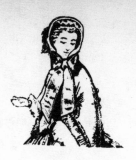

Raspberry (Rubus idaeus). It is claimed to take of a concoction made from the leaves of this plant shall diminish if not wholly banish the pains of childbearing, a vinegar concocted from this plant is used to bring down fevers and relieve colds.

Rattle, Red (Pedicularis palustris). It is said an infusion of this plant in wine would give lift to humours. Also recommended as a safeguard against many disorders of mens' systems.

Rowan (Sorbus aucuparia). This tree is more commonly known as mountain ash. A concoction made from the berries of this tree, rich in vitamin C, was at one time widely used to prevent and cure scurvy.

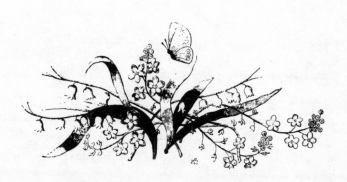

Sainfoin (Onobrychis viciifolia). Infusions of this plant were given to nursing mothers to enhance the richness and flow of their milk, also claimed to be a cure for diseases of the bladder.

Samphire, Rock (Crithmum maritimum). A plant that is said to dispel indigestion.

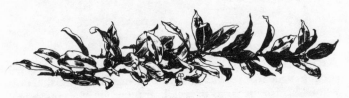

Sanicle (Sanicula europaea). This plant has been held in high esteem through the ages, it is said to cure all hurts or wounds internal or external should you take of its juices.

Saxifrage, Burnet (Pimpinella saxifraga). Herbalists used a concoction from the leaves and stems to heal wounds and stop bleeding.

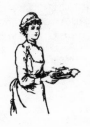

Saxifrage, Meadow (Saxifraga granulata). Said to rid the gallstone.

Saxifrage, Opposite Leaved Golden (Chrysosplenium oppositifolium). Used to rid any disease of the spleen.

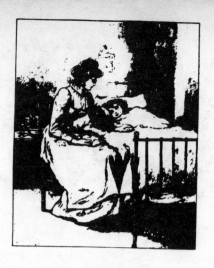

Scabious, Devil's Bit (Succisa pratensis). This plant, apart from its healing abilities for skin complaints, was used to cure sore throats and reckoned to be an antidote for snake bites.

Scabious, Field (Knautia arvensis). A concoction made of this plant was used in the same way as small scabious and devil's bit scabious, to cure skin complaints.

Scabious, Small (Scabiosa columbaria). Said to cure the itch and many diseases of the skin; also used to cure wounds – for this the juice of the plant was recommended.

Selfheal (Prunella vulgaris). It is written that an early Greek physician used infusions made from this plant to cure tonsillitis and other complaints of the throat.

Silverweed (Potentilla anserina). Another plant much used to arrest throat infections. Another use was to stem the flow of blood from a wound.

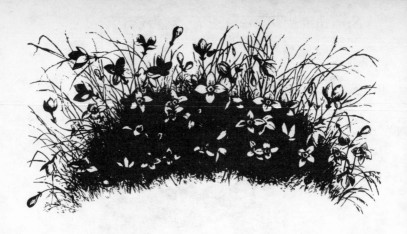

Skullcap (Scutellaria galericulata). Herbalists dried and powdered this plant. Should one suffer nervous tension, hysteria or St. Vitus' Dance the order would be to infuse a small amount of this powder in boiling water. As this is a very potent drug it must never be used in large quantities or the patient will have adverse results to those wanted. Use with caution.

Sneezewort (Achillea ptarmica). To chew of the root of this plant was claimed to rid toothache sufferers of all pain.

Soapwort (Saponaria officinalis). The lather given off by the greenery of this plant when boiled was recommended by herbalists as a medicinal shampoo to strengthen delicate hair. Not to be taken internally.

Solomon's Seal (Polygonatum multiflorum). The medicinal properties of this plant have been known for hundreds of years. It is claimed to be able to seal and heal wounds, mend broken bones and its roots, when crushed and made into a poultice, will cure bruises.

Speedwell, Common (Veronica officinalis). Used to cure a host of ills, including leprosy.

Spurge, Petty (Euphorbia peplus). A plant that warrants caution when used because of its poisonous properties. Herbalists used the juice of the plant to burn off warts and corns.

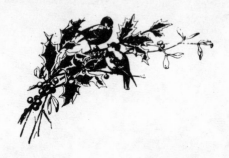

Stitchwort, Greater (Stellaria holostea). To relieve the stitch herbalists used a concoction obtained by mixing crushed acorns with a fusion made from this plant.

Sumac, Stag's Horn (Rhus typhina). A concoction obtained from the roots of this tree was at one time used to control and break fevers.

Sundew, Round Leaved (Drosera rotundifolia). Another plant used for the burning off of warts and corns, herbalists used the dew-like droplets that gathered on its leaves for this purpose. The plant was also reckoned to be a stimulant to cattle at breeding times, said to raise their sexual desires.

Tamarisk (Tamarix anglica). An infusion made from this shrub was at one time highly recommended as a general pick-you-up tonic, also reckoned to cure rheumatism and ease bruises.

Tansy (Tanacetum vulgare). Claimed to extend the life of those that drank of an infusion of this plant. Also said to prevent miscarriage.

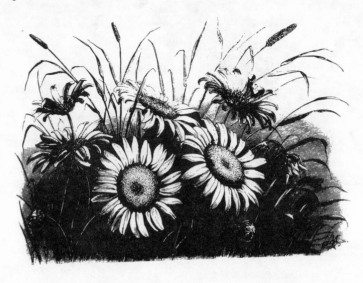

Thistle, Cotton (Onopordon acanthium). This plant it is claimed cures cancer, tension and bone disorders.

Thistle, Melancholy (Cirsium helenium). It was claimed that if an infusion of the leaves of this plant were taken, it dispelled all sadness, the fusion to be done with wine.

Thyme (Thymus praecox). The oil of this plant is useful because of its antiseptic content, this giving it healing potential.

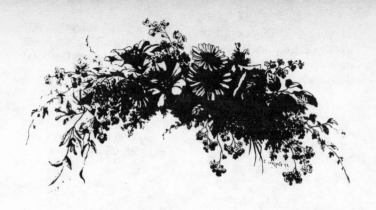

Tormentil (Potentilla erecta). 'Suffer not the pains of toothache, take of the crushed roots of this plant and such pains shall be banished.'

Tutsan (Hypericum androsaemum). There is much to be said of the healing qualities of this plant, the leaves were used to cure cuts and gashes, sometimes of a very severe nature.

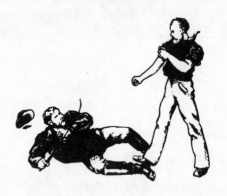

Valerian, Common (Valeriana officinalis). Juices obtained from the roots of this plant have been used for many years to calm those in shock, also to sedate those of an aggressive nature.

Vervain (Verbena officinalis). Apothecaries thought very highly of this plant because of its medicinal benefits, and often used it as a preventative medicine against many types of diseases.

Vetch, Kidney (Anthyllis vulneraria). Widely used as a cure for cuts and grazes, said to speedily heal them, it was also claimed that this plant was able to put right kidney disorders.

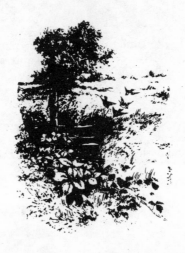

Wall Pellitory (Parietaria diffusa). Fear not the loss of shoulder length locks. Take of the juice of this plant fused with honey and they will be yours forever.

Watercress (Nasturtium officinale). Reckoned to be good for cleansing of the blood, also rich in vitamin C.

Watercress, Fools' (Apium nodiflorum). A decoction of this plant and other watercress was said to be good for those dieting.

Water Lily, White (Nymphaea alba). The oils obtained from this plant were held in high esteem by herbalists, and was used by them to cure baldness as well as many womanly ills.

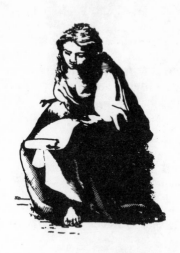

Water Parsnip, Lesser (Berula erecta). Take of the roots of this plant and boil in vinegar, use then as a poultice to rid any swelling or inflammation. Should an old sore be persistent the same concoction can be used to cleanse and will promote healing.

Wild Service Tree (Sorbus torminalis). The fruit of this tree has long been used to cure those suffering dysentery, also recommended for those complaining of colic.

Winter Cress, Common (Barbarea vulgaris). Much used by those caring for the casualties of early gun battles, they would take of the leaves of this plant to cover the open wounds.

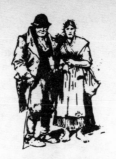

Wintergreen, Chickweed (Trientalis europaea). It was said this plant had the ability to cure blood poisoning and was used for this purpose by herbalists, also used by them to heal wounds.

Wintergreen, Common (Pyrola minor). Should the oil that is obtained from the leaves of this plant be rubbed upon any part of the body that aches, it is reckoned that those aches shall be banished. The leaves are also recommended as a healant for cuts and to staunch bleeding.

Woodsage (Teucrium scorodonia). Take and dry this plant's leaves then infuse as tea. This it was said, would protect you from rheumatism.

Woundwort, Marsh (Stachys palustris). To bind the leaves of this plant, even on the deepest wound, will heal it very quickly.

Yarrow (Achillea millefolium). Said to be capable of cleansing the deepest wounds and curing even the most gruesome injuries obtained in battles of yesteryear.

Yellow Wort (Blackstonia perfoliata). 'Suffer not with a bad temper, be this your problem then take of this plant and that temper shall no longer plague you.'

PART THREE

STORIES OF
GRANDMOTHER'S CURES

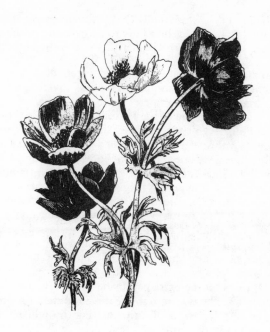

Warding Off Colds

Every Winter when I was a little girl, my mother put a block
of camphor in a small bag and tied it around my neck. I wore
it from November until May. The camphor was renewed
when it was wasted away. I still wear a block of camphor
which I put inside my bra, and I never have a cold.

Miss A.H. Bolton, Lancs.

91

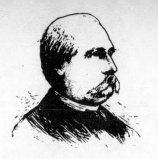

Backache

I thought you might be interested in an old remedy for
backache and pains in the hip. This was given to my great
grandfather, who was a horse trader, by a vet of all people,
many years ago at one of the horsefairs he attended. I expect
even if you haven't seen one of these horsefairs you have
heard of them. My grandfather had a string of six fine horses
to sell on this day, but was fearful he wasn't going to be able
to, for those interested in buying would most certainly wish
to see them trot, and he was plagued with a terrible back pain.
That is until he explained his plight to a vet, who rather
casually said 'You know, were we to watch the ways of other
animals, we would not suffer many of the ills and pains we
do. Take your back problem – had you stretched on leaving
your bed to ensure that fluid, built up between the many
joints overnight was removed, the disc that has obviously
slipped, (because the extra gap made by this fluid) could not
have slipped. The way to remove it is to stretch, so forcing it
out; this is in fact what all other animals do whenever they
rouse. Follow this rule and backache will be banished.
Method: stand with feet about eighteen inches apart, place
palms of hands on hips then lean back alternating from the left
and right. To relieve aching hip sit on the floor, open your
legs approximately four feet, push forward as far as possible,
repeat four or five times, and then do same on the right leg.
The pain will go, repeat if pain returns.' My great grandfather
passed this advice onto his children and they to theirs. Thank-
fully my mother gave me this advice, it has proved to be
sound, for I in my ninety-third year have never suffered with
backache.

Miss L.A. Burgess, Birmingham

Acne and Tension

Hearing you were writing a book on old cures, prompted me to write, thinking two, given to me as a student nurse years ago, by an old dear, might be of interest to you. I suffered terrible acne, the pimples just would not go, they continually wept and spread, so much so that I was too embarrassed to socialise at all. Unbeknown to me this old dear must have noted my plight, for as I straightened her bed just after visiting hours she drew my attention to a pot plant that her husband had left and said, 'That is for you my love.' I thanked her, but explained I was not one for gardening. She smiled, and said, 'No matter dear, for when you have used the leaves of this one, I will get Hubby to bring another, and we will do that until those pimples are removed completely.' Seeing I was still bemused she explained in more detail. 'After washing, you take one of the iceplant's leaves and break a piece off, then just rub the open ends of the leaves upon the spots. After a while you will find they will go.' At this I chuckled, for if what the old lady told me was so, why didn't doctors recommend it? She seemingly read my mind, 'Modern medicine is too wrapped up in itself my dear, and sometimes don't see what is directly beneath their noses. Perhaps another reason is who would buy all those modern ointments if it was made known this simple plant would cure?' Deciding there was logic in what she said I decided to give it a try. Result, within two weeks my face was free of pimples and for the past fifty years I have ensured that I have at least half a dozen iceplants in the house, for I have found they are also fantastic for curing cuts, grazes and cold sores.

The other cure this dear old lady gave me was for tension, she noticed my tenseness when I was sitting my exams. One day she beckoned me to her bed and as I approached, she took from her locker beside the bed a brown paper bag. This she handed to me saying, 'When feeling tense dear, just breathe into the bag, ensure you breathe back that air you breathed out, do this for about thirty seconds, and your tension will go!'

Mrs. D. Curtis-Hayward, Wilts.

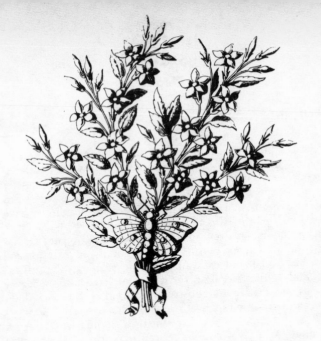

Diarrhoea

I thought you might like to hear of the uses of tincture of red lavenders. This is a very old and wonderful cure for diarrhoea, but almost impossible to procure except at very old fashioned chemists. I was brought up on it, my mother being a confirmed homeopathist who worked under the direction of Dr. Shackleton, father of the famous Sir Ernest. Red lavender used to be given as much as could be absorbed on a lump of sugar, the results were marvellous. My brother, in Calcutta, used it with camphor to cure his Indian servants with cholera.

Mrs. D. Curtis-Hayward, Wilts.

'Miracle Brew' for Baldness and Ageing

Miracle Brew from an old grandmother's recipe. Eighty years old, Mrs. Samual Jeoyler of Istianth, frail and toothless, was recommended to try it for getting younger. After she did, she grew hair on her head and was able to walk five miles to collect a new set of false teeth and felt younger, fit and well. The doctors were staggered and said it was a miracle of faith.

Mrs. D. Curtis-Hayward, Wilts.

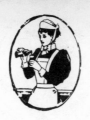

Cuts and Open Wounds

When I was a child in my native Yorkshire, it was the custom in addition to making mince pies at Christmas to make lots of Yorkshire cheesecakes (sometimes called curd tarts). Some of these were saved and left to go mouldy. Pieces of the very mouldy tarts were rubbed upon any open cuts whether minor or serious, and a very effective cure this was too. I think it must have been the forerunner of penicillin. The tarts were made by creaming together ¼lb butter, 3oz sugar, add ½lb curd, 3oz currants, 1 tablespoon flour and 2 beaten eggs. Flavour with nutmeg, mix well and bake in quick oven.

Mrs. J. Baxter, Dyfed

Loss of Hair and Eczema

Sixty years ago I knew a housekeeper at a nursing home near to where I lived. She had her mother staying with her, who was well into her seventies. She looked her age, except for her hair, this was a shimmering black and beautiful. She told us that when in her youth, she contracted eczema in her hair, face and arms, and was really in a bad state. Her hair fell out and became very thin and lank. A gypsy called at her home and could not help but notice her plight. She advised her to dig up some burdock roots and stew them, strain off the water and drink a small wineglass full every morning for nine days, leave for nine days then repeat. After three months of this treatment she was better, her hair that had been very thin began to grow again, and in fact to the day she died it was as black as ebony.

Mrs. E. Hall, Shropshire

Impetigo

When I was three years old, I suffered a bad attack of impetigo. My face was in a dreadful state, smothered in scabs and the Doctor gave mother some red greasy ointment; she was instructed to first bathe my face to soften the scabs and then apply the ointment. This did no good at all and if anything, was getting worse. An old lady that lived nearby advised my mother to dust the scabs with flowers of sulphur. Within a week of this treatment my face was much better, the scabs dried up and simply dropped off without the awful picking. I have always ensured to keep flowers of sulphur in the house, and when my own children had mild attacks of impetigo I used it with the same results, no need to visit the doctor.

Mrs. H. Williams, Shrewsbury

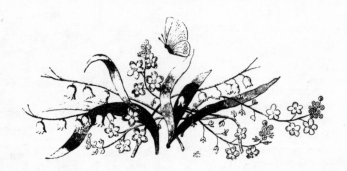

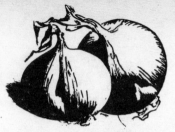

Sore Throat and Chilblains

In answer to your request for old remedies, I well remember if my sister or I developed a sore throat, my mother would get Dad to bring in the largest onion. These normally, at the time of the year when sore throats and coughs were rampant, would be beautifully strung up in the garden shed. She would peel it, and cut it half horizontally, then place each half, cut side upwards, in a deep saucer, puting onto the cut edges of the onion as much demerara sugar as would go. This she would leave to stand all night, or day as the case might be – in other words about twelve hours. Next night or morning the saucers would be full of juice that had come from the onion and sugar. Of this mother would give us two spoonsful before we went to bed, and a further two before going out into the cold morning air for school. This reminds me of another cure. One of my brothers and a sister suffered the most awful chilblains on their hands. We all lived in a small village, mid Hampshire; the cottage we lived in had no indoor lavatory, so at night we would use pots under the bed. Well, my brother and sister were made to soak their chilblained hands every morning in their own cold urine before leaving for school. They were not allowed to wash their hands after soaking them, mother insisted they let them dry naturally. Can you imagine the smell in the classroom, what with our onion breath, and to top that my brother and sister's smelly hands. It was awful.

Mrs. E.L. Park, Southampton

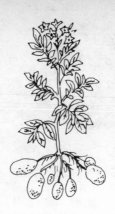

Health Tonic

My grandfather's recipe for good health was to chop up an onion with a handful of parsley, boil it in rough cider and sweeten with honey. He boiled this liquid and had two teaspoonfuls every night. He lived to be 101; he might have been alive today if he had not been knocked down by a child riding a bicycle.

Mrs. D. Tilbrook, Essex

Sore Throat

When I was a child, and had a sore throat my mother put a rasher of bacon round my throat at bedtime, or a sock that I had been wearing. Now that bacon is so dear I settle for my tights around my neck, that gives me relief.

Mrs. N. Hale, Berks.

Quinsy

A potato baked in its jacket dropped in a sock and put hot around the neck is very good. I did this to a friend who was in agony with a quinsy and it had burst by morning, much to her relief.

Mrs. M. Hale, Berks.

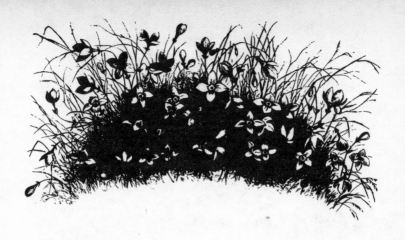

Carbuncles

The following may interest you. Around 1920, when I was a young girl, my father suffered half a dozen carbuncles in quick succession. An old fellow, engaged on painting our house, sympathised with my father and remarked that 'We didn't 'ave none of them in the Navy.' My father replied that he supposed this was due to the antiseptic qualities of the salt air and the painter said that the cure was to suck a nutmeg until it disappeared. Afterwards my father laughed this to scorn as another 'old wives tale', but mother looked a little thoughtful and advised him to try this, as it might prove more beneficial than it appeared. Father, still scoffing, finally agreed to do so and surprise, surprise, no more carbuncles. The sequel came many years later, when during the war I was in contact with a poor woman who was suffering from this painful complaint. In fact she had had over thirty carbuncles despite medical treatment. The war ended and I did not meet her again until five years later and upon enquiring about the carbuncles, she said that she had been free from them for the past two or three years, but was still under medical care and observation and had to watch her diet. She reeled off a list of things from which she was barred, but added some that she had to take, amongst the latter a stipulated quantity of freshly ground nutmeg each day! The old sailor-turned-painter/decorator was neither a Welshman nor a Grandmother, but certainly seems to have proved the efficiency of yet another 'old wives cure'.

Mrs. E.W. Hatton, Dyfed

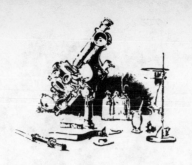

Whooping Cough and Shingles

We are so used to modern high pressure drugs and National Health prescriptions that it seems impossible to us that so recently as the last century incantations and herbal dosage, to say nothing of simples and brews were still the order of the day in many rural areas. Visiting the West Country I chatted with an old gentleman who knew a 'wise woman' in his boyhood and remembered the days when sick folk travelled far to get the right remedy be it word, action or treatment. Like the Son of Sirach, the country bred folk insisted 'with many cures for confirmation' that 'The Lord hath created medicines out of the earth', and he that is wise will not abhor (disapprove of) them. In the practice of 'country treatment' there was much that was, and is, basically sound, though there was even more that was undoubtedly quackery. It was believed for instance that a page of the Bible eaten between bread and butter was a cure for fits; while for whooping cough the patient's relatives were told to cut a hair from a donkey's back, where the cross appears, and place in a silken bag to be hung round the sufferers neck. Persons suffering from shingles were advised to scrape the koom (verdigris) from a church bell and apply as an ointment. There is of course, another side of country cures and not all are to be dismissed as readily as should the foregone. Many truly herbal remedies are passed down in a tradition of healing, and John Evelyn was not far from the truth when he said 'If the medicinal properties of the leaves, bark, berries etc., were thoroughly known I cannot tell what our countrymen would ail for which he might not find a remedy from every hedge, either for sickness or wound.'

Reverend W. Fancutt, Isle of Wight

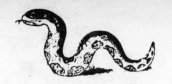

Septic Cuts

I expect you know that snakes shed their skins (slough) every spring, and mystery concerns the use of these skins, and I assure you it is absolutely true. It happened some eighty years ago, almost (that will give my age away). One of my sisters had a very bad finger, it had turned septic and was oozing pus. One day as mother was dressing her, a gypsy woman came selling the usual things. My sister followed Mother when she answered the door and the old gypsy noticed her poisoned finger. 'That's a nasty mess you have there my dear, I will soon put that better,' she said. With this she removed her hat, and from the lining she drew a small package. Undoing this she took from it a piece of snakeskin, this she gave Mother, then instructed that she must wrap this around the child's finger and then bandage it up. My sister didn't want a piece of snake put on her finger first off, but in the end gave in to Mother's wishes. Sure enough within a day or two her finger was quite well again.

Mrs. A.L. Baker, South Devon

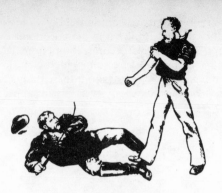

Strained Joints, Sprains and Bruises

My experience of the value of malt vinegar began over fifty years ago when I was treating a horse for sprained fetlock, and was advised by an elderly gypsy to use bandages soaked in malt vinegar (the stronger the better). The result was amazing – it reduced the inflammation and swelling in less than a week, and I found it equally effective on subsequent occasions. At that time, I myself was an active gymnast, an activity which resulted frequently in strained joints and muscles and incurred serious expense for embrocation (which itself contains a high proportion of vinegar). In view of my success with animal treatment, I decided to substitute the use of malt vinegar bandages and the results were beyond my expectation, especially how quickly it withdrew the inflammation and bruising of any injured limb. It must definitely be *malt* vinegar and I keep bandages well soaked.

Mr. C. Watts, Southampton

Warts and Stutters

A few years back a very old lady born and bred in North Bovey, told me that as a little girl a gypsy woman called at their cottage and noticed that she had several warts on her hands and that her younger sister had a bad stutter. She prescribed the following cures. For the warts: brush them with an elderberry flower, throw the flower over the left shoulder, but under no circumstances look where it falls.

For the stutter: brew a strong solution of ivy leaves and with a cloth soaked in the infusion, bathe the outside of the throat. Both children had complete cures. Sometime later I was cutting a hedge and there were some elderberry flowers and although being slightly sceptical about these things decided to have a go; a few weeks later my wart just disappeared.

F.F. Radford, Devon

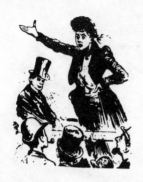

Obstinate Cough

I have a letter written by my grandfather, Oliver George Marling, to his sister around a hundred years ago. It is not dated but they both died in 1892.

Dear Eliza,
I forgot to send you this recipe when I wrote on Saturday. It was given by Lady Fitzharding to Miss Pearce as coming from the first physicians (sic) to London. Make a strong solution of saltpetre dissolved in water, get a clean sheet of white blotting paper, thoroughly soak it then make the paper quite dry. Cut off a piece and put it into a plate, set fire to one corner (it will burn like touch paper). Let the patient inhale the smoke holding the mouth open over the plate and drawing it in, it should be done sitting up in bed and last thing. White blotting paper is named because nothing injurious is in the making thereof. It is simple and might be of use though I hope you are finding all such on the decrease. With best love in great haste, Yours etc., ever Oliver.

There is no evidence of its efficiency, nor have I tried it myself.

K.C. Marling, Herefordshire

Whooping Cough

In 1920 at the age of two I had whooping cough. Having
exhausted all popular remedies my mother was instructed by
my grandmother to trap two mice, which apparently were
abundant in our house. Having procured the two mice my
mother prepared them as one would a rabbit, and baked
them. I ate them with great relish by all accounts. My mother
told me in later years that my whooping cough was cured in
about two days.

Mrs. A.E. Gould, Salisbury

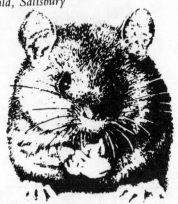

Weak and Twisted Legs

I recall my late mother (who would have been ninety-nine
this year) telling me that when one of her elder brothers was
very young, I should think about eighteen months old, his
legs were so weak and twisted (I think they were called
bowed) he just could not stand up. An old gypsy lady called
selling pegs, she asked what ailed the child. Grannie showed
her the baby's legs. The old gypsy told her to ask her husband
to get up early in the morning and collect all the snails he
could find, put them in a muslin bag and the slime that
dripped through she was to rub into the baby's legs. She was
to do this every day until his legs were all right. Grandad got
up early as instructed and collected the snails and Grandmother rubbed the slime onto the baby's legs (Uncle Harry).
He gradually improved, eventually he was able to run about,
he never had any more trouble with his legs and lived well
into his seventies. Perhaps it was the continual massage that
rectified his deformed legs – Grandmother was sure of one
thing, her hands had never been so soft before!

Miss P.M. Worthington, Southampton

Quinsy

After Mother married in 1907 she suffered continual attacks of quinsy. My parents lived at a village shop; an old gypsy lady called into the shop to purchase some groceries, she asked what was wrong with my mother's throat, on being told she pointed to a side of bacon and said 'Cut that piece of rusty bacon off and tie it around the lady's neck when she goes to bed tonight, put the rusty part towards her skin.' By 'the rusty part' she was referring to the rind that had been browned when smoked to preserve it. Daddy asked mother at bedtime if she was going to do as the gypsy had said. My mother remembered how well the snail cure had worked and decided she would. It appears that during the night her throat got hotter and hotter, the fat on the bacon melted, made a greasy mess and smelt horrible, but before the morning the quinsy broke, and she never had another attack.

Miss P.M. Worthington, Southampton

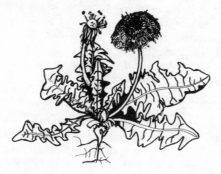

Sinus Trouble

I frequently had severe attacks of sinus infection causing intolerable pain, and was advised a surgical operation would be necessary if it continued. One night following the use of a menthol ointment, I was troubled with nasal irritation, and camphorated oil was the only thing I was able to find to give me relief. I placed a small quantity up each nostril and in addition to relief of irritation, after a short period it freed the mucus obstructing the sinus. Following this experience when I had further attacks I reverted to the use of the oil, and after several attacks I used it nightly when retiring, and the attacks came less frequently and ceased completely after about six months.

Mr. C. Watts, Southampton

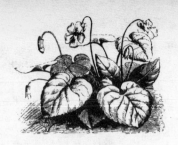

Colic and Melancholy

Reading of your interest in old remedies brought to mind one both my mother and grandmother swore by regarding its medicinal properties. The story goes: my grandfather suffered colic many years – this it can only be assumed made him very ill tempered, at times he was intolerable and almost impossible to live with – no matter who visited, he would be so abrupt and rude to them, as the years passed those that knew didn't visit and grandmother lost many friends. One day an old gypsy called selling her wares, Grandma rushed to the door on hearing the knock, fearful that Grandad would get there first and inevitably be rude to the visitor. 'Buy some pegs me dear,' the gypsy said as soon as grandmother opened the door. Grandma looked nervously down the garden, the fear in her eyes slowly going as she noted Grandad was working in the vegetable patch and had not seen, nor heard, the gypsy enter. The gypsy noted Grandma's nervousness, and attributed it to her. 'Ere I ant gonna rob yu lady, yu don aff tu worry.' Grandmother apologetically explained to the gypsy the reason for her nervousness. The gypsy after listening attentively to grandmother's tale of woe, smilingly asked, 'Would you be interested in a cure fer 'is colic and 'is sour nature?' Grandmother's reply was one of hopelessness. 'If only there were such a cure,' she sighed. 'Cross me 'and wiv silver lady, and a cure fer colic an' the grumps will be yours,' the gypsy replied. For many days grandmother did as the wise old gypsy had advised, and sure enough grandad stopped complaining of colic. What was even more unbelievable his temperament became so placid and easy going it was hard to believe he was the same person, now he was so pleasant to everyone. The cure was simple: cabbage, cooked with honey and salt added to it, so simple yet so effective, used for many years by such great cultures as the Greek, Egyptian and the Roman.

Mrs. J. Snelgrove, Hants.

Inflammation of the Eye, Boils and Infected Cuts

Re your interest in Grandmother's Cures. The two I have in mind were passed from my Grandmother (1872–1914). The first was known as 'Eyewater' for inflammation of the eyes, and was just a dilute solution of zinc sulphate. Eye droppers were unknown to the old folk – they used a teaspoon. I cannot give the strength of the solution as I never saw it in writing. I sadly do not remember my Grandmother, my mother (1892–1957) passed them on to me. The other was ointment which had some local renown in treating boils and infected cuts, again I cannot give quantities, but as a boy in the early twenties I saw it made. Leaf lard from the butcher was rendered slowly to avoid burning. The clear fat was poured into a pan and over gentle heat were added bits of beeswax and a substance called burgundy pitch which was rather like the beeswax in appearance, but darker with a reddish tinge. When the mixture was uniformly mixed it was poured into a jar. A few people who remember my grandmother tell how they used to call and purchase three penny boxes of the ointment. The last regular user was an old bricklayer who had a box every weekend for his chapped hands.

Mr. W. Feeney, Lancs.

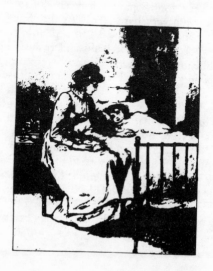

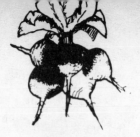

Hay Fever

During the very hot summer of 1959 I was badly affected with asthma, after an attack of hayfever, my third son having been born in the February of the same year. At that time an elderly aunt of my husband's side of the family produced an old handwritten recipe book, this had been handed down in the family. It was from this I acquired the remedy for hayfever. The aunt said it had cured an old uncle; I tried it and it most definitely cured me. The recipe read: one tablespoon of *lime water* – not lime juice or cordial. The lime water to be taken in a wineglass of milk, three times daily. Preferably start treatment prior to the time of year hay fever usually attacks the patient.

Mrs. V. Milford, Hants.

Gashes and Bleeding and Coughs

Your letter in the paper interested me greatly. I am sixty-six years old, or will be next March, and I recall very clearly when I was very young, having a severe fall and bashing my forehead on some very hard steps. At the time I was in the care of my grandmother, and I can remember very vividly how she grabbed me by the hand and rushed me to an old outhouse. She grabbed a handful of cobwebs down from one of the walls and smothered my face and profusely bleeding wound with these cobwebs. The gaping wound healed up beautifully. It is an experience I have never forgotten. I also recall that my father had his own special cure i.e. cobwebs wax. Splinters were always cleanly extracted by a dab of this wax; firstly heated on a candle and dropped on the splinter. This he would also use on any nasty gashes from falling on gravel etc., it stung for a moment at first, but always healed the wound beautifully. A good old fashioned cough syrup my mother used was grated onions and carrots mixed with brown sugar, left to stand overnight – the juice was delicious and healing.

Mrs. D. Le Mercier, Jersey

Whooping Cough

I was very interested *re* your article on folklore remedies. My daughter who now lives in Crawley, contracted whooping cough at an early age. I was beside myself and had no idea as to what I should do to relieve the baby's plight, that was until one of my neighbours gave me a cure that had been given to her by her mother. The instructions were – slice a turnip and swede, put down first a layer of turnip in a deepish bowl, cover this with sugar, place a layer of swede onto this, sprinkle a further layer of sugar, continue doing this until swede and turnip are used. Leave for twenty-four hours, this produced a liquid and it was this my neighbour told me to give my child. I did and it resulted in her immediate relief, and I might add mine as well.

Mrs. E. Loveridge, Southampton

Fever

My grandmother used to travel around quite a lot, and at one time one of her sons took ill, much to Gran's disgust a doctor had to come. He told Gran that her son had pneumonia and was in a very bad way, did not think he would pull through and he could do very little for him since he had such a fever, but would call and see him next day. My gran now knowing what was wrong, did no more than go to the nearest village butcher's shop and here bought two melts (they are like big pieces of liver) and they had to be fresh. When she got back to her son, these melts were tied on the bottom of his feet and left there until the next day. By that time the smell in their caravan was awful, as the melts had rotted, but her son was better and all the fever had gone.

When the Doctor came he couldn't believe it was the same boy he had seen the day before and asked Gran what she had done. She took off the melts and showed them to the Doctor, they were black and had drawn the fever down into the melts and cured her son. The Doctor was amazed and asked why had she called him out if she knew what to do. Gran told him she only wanted to know what was the matter with her son. That son lived until he was seventy-six and died in 1970.

Mrs. G. Liniham, Hants.

Warts, Bunions, Verruca and Alopecia

I am a retired Prison Officer, and through the years have picked up a few remedies that although could not be called Grandmother's Cures, for I have gathered them in the main from gypsies I have met from time to time during my service, they are old time cures and they all work. First the cure for warts. Steal a piece of raw meat, rub it on the wart, or warts, bury the meat and as this rots away so the warts will disappear – approximately five to six weeks. We had a friend whose young son had warts from head to foot, he had been treated by a doctor to no effect. Finally I persuaded his mother to try my cure and hey presto! all the warts disappeared. I have since cured many people, in fact never having a failure. My wife at one time suffered with a very painful bunion. While out one day with a working party of prisoners, I asked a gypsy convict if he knew of a cure for bunions. 'Oh yes, simple,' he said. 'Meatsfoot oil.' I asked him where I might get it. He said from any chemist or leather shop. I bought some from Boots, it cost sixpence. Each night and morning I rubbed a little on the bunion, sure enough it slowly shrunk and the pain disappeared. I have since cured several people with the same remedy. By the way I am sure that gypsies know the cure for baldness, the reason I believe this is I can't ever in my life remember seeing a bald gypsy.

The verruca, or many headed corn. My daughter suffered one of these infectious afflictions but after repeated treatment from a Doctor with no success, an elderly lady told my wife that a simple old cure was to wet a knob of soda and rub it onto the verucca night and morning. The many headed corn disappeared in a few days. Next falling hair, this is called Alopecia. The hair falls out leaving large bald patches – an old barber told me of a cure for this disease. Just rub gas water onto it. Gas water – this was the water through which coal gas was passed during purification and could be obtained for nothing from the old gasworks. The barber gave me some, he kept a supply in a carboy. I used it and rid myself of this complaint, and also recommended it to many other people. Of course now in the days of North Sea Gas the end of coal gasworks, it is now unobtainable.

Mr. E. Goody, Hants.

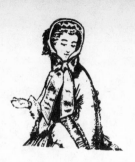

Swollen Knee

My father was transferred from Belfast at the start of World War I and my mum brought us four children over. The only place she could get for us to live, for a short time as she thought then, was in the poor district of Bootle, near the docks, as my dad was at Harland & Wolfe shipyard. The people living near us were all very illiterate, each family had stacks of children, so of course the women thought my mum was 'posh' and educated, and used to come to her with their problems. My mum used to even deliver their babies before the midwife could arrive. Well one person, Mrs. Carr, came to our house in a terrible state, crying and terrified, lifted her 'Mary Ellen' skirt up to show Mum her knee, which was the size of a football and red and angry looking, and very painful.

Seems the doctor had tried and just could not do anymore, so had sent her along to the Bootle Hospital, where they told her she had to go in the following week for an operation. As you can imagine, in those days, hospital was enough to scare anyone, but an operation, that was even worse and her with a houseful of kids. We used to go to a dairy yard near the docks for our milk, take a jug and the milk was served from a churn, and I can always remember a few cows round the backyard, so it seems my mum went there next day and asked for some cow dung, I think at that time they thought she was mad, because she didn't give any explanation why she wanted it. My brother and I came home from school and the smell that met us was awful, the whole house reeked with it. At the time we had no idea why until we went into the kitchen and there was our mum with a shovel of the cow dung on a red hot fire, holding the shovel over the fire to roast this stuff, and when it was steaming she threw it quickly into a clean pillow case and ran like hell past us and down the street to poor Mrs. Carr's house (we found out after), to put it on the bad knee. This she did again that evening and I believe for the next few days, it's a wonder my dad didn't throw her out, the house was terrible with the smell. We didn't know at the time what she was doing. Anyway next week Mrs. Carr went to hospital as arranged, and was back home within an hour or so. The doctors couldn't believe what they saw: the knee was the same shape as her other one, nor a mark nor a pain or anything, can you imagine the smug look on our Mum's face?

Mrs. R. Woodland, Clwyd

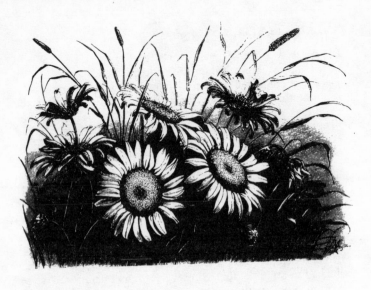

Whitlows and Whooping Cough

About 1935 I had a bad whitlow on my thumb. I went to stay with friends in Switzerland, who on seeing my ailment immediately from the medicine cupboard produced a jar of lily of the valley leaves in brandy. My thumb was wrapped in a leaf, in a short time – two days – complete cure. I was told it had to be lily of the valley but have often wondered if the brandy was really the operative ingredient. The cure for whooping cough is purely hearsay, but on reliable authority. Working in Westmorland 1931–1934 in a number of villages, children with whooping cough had a mole skin tied around the neck.

Miss M.E. Andrews, Hants.

Cuts

My great grandmother (born 1914) was brought up on a farm and became a farmer's wife. Whenever a bad gash was sustained – and farm implements could give nasty deep cuts, and very unhygenic ones – she always applied the mouldy jam top directly onto the wound before bandaging.

Miss Petrie, East Sussex

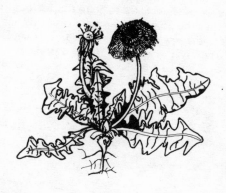

Warts

When I was a young girl at school, many years ago – I am now seventy-seven – I remember the number of children that had big ugly warts on their hands. The other children would not take hold of their hands in games. We had no money in those days to buy things from the chemist's shop; we were told to pluck the dandelion flower when in full bloom, the thick white liquid that came from it was to be rubbed onto the wart, we were to do this for several days as frequently as possible. This we did and were delighted when the warts vanished.

Miss Petrie, East Sussex

Constipation and Cuts

It is a great pleasure to write to you, as so many people doubt the old remedies, or what the gypsies said, but I found them very helpful. One told me to give my young children a teaspoon of castor oil as a cure for constipation. I have also found castor oil unbeatable for cuts of any description. In my cupboard I have always kept three kinds of oil in case of mishap: camphor, olive and castor. I remember one such mishap: our shopkeeper fell and gashed the side of her head. The cut looked terrible, about two and a half inches long and very deep, even so she refused to go to the doctors and have it stitched. I stuck the gash together with castor oil and covered with a plaster, there was none more surprised than I when the plaster was removed and not a mark was there. The same thing happened when my daughter's finger was almost severed, I stuck it back on smothering it with castor oil, it healed and you can see no mark. Because of these facts and that they actually happened to me, I have great faith in the things I have tried.

Mrs. M. Carter, Hants.

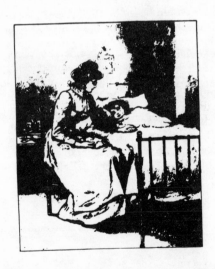

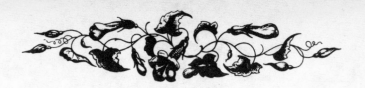

Warts and Whooping Cough

As a child (I am a widow in my early sixties) I had warts on my fingers and could not get rid of them. My aged grandmother, in the Island of Islay, told me to squeeze the white milk out of the stem of a dandelion on to them or to spit on them first thing in the morning (something in my morning spittle). Being desperate, I did both and the warts vanished without trace. Many years later, just after the last war, my children had whooping cough very badly (unheard of today) and were subject to most distressing and sustained fits of coughing. At the time an elderly widow from Australia was staying with us. She told me how her son (who had been killed in the RAAF) had been similarly afflicted as a little boy. In the streets of Melbourne he had taken a very bad bout of coughing (this would be in the 1920's) and a stranger stopped and told his mother to use this old remedy. Take a new laid (essential) egg and cover it with vinegar for twenty-four hours. The shell dissolves in the vinegar. To this liquid add honey and melt over heat. The mixture must then be stirred with a *red hot* poker. A few spoonsful will cure the worst cough. Well, I was desperate so I tried it. Living in a modern centrally heated flat it was difficult to get a red hot poker. The egg was easy as there were farms around. I managed to heat a hot poker in my incinerator and it worked – the desperate coughing bouts ceased!

Mrs. E.A. Smith, Scotland

115

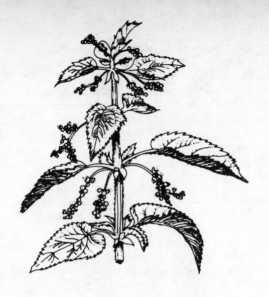

Blood purifier

My Granny Ings was New Forest born and bred, and she knew all the many lovely herbs that grew there. Sadly I can't remember the names of all those that she collected, but I do know of two useful ones, woodsage and wormwood. At the appropriate time of the year, Granny would gather these herbs in great quantities and hang them in the outhouse to dry, she would then take them to Ringwood and sell them to the various chemists, who would use them to make up all sorts of medicines and ointments. One large bunch of woodsage and another of wormwood always found its way to our house every winter. Mother would put some of the dried herbs into a large jug, pour boiling water onto them and the next morning we children were given an eggcupful before setting off for school. I remember it tasted very bitter, but we were used to it so drank it without any qualms. Mother said it was to purify the blood, whether it did or not I don't know, we were certainly a pretty healthy bunch of children.

Mrs. R. Jacobs, Hants.

Nettlerash and Wasp Stings

When I was a youngster if I were to eat rhubarb or strawberries, immediately after I would break out in a nettlerash. Granny's cure was to boil some young nettle tops then drink the liquid. This treatment was only necessary once, since treatment as a child I have never suffered these ill effects. Eating an apple one day, unhappily for me a wasp had decided to make a meal of the same apple. His reaction when I took a bite at the piece he was upon was instant, a sting for me in the mouth. Granny's cure: suck a raw onion, this stopped the swelling, and in my case most certainly eased the pain.

Mrs. R. Jacobs, Hants.

Blood Poisoning

Many years ago when I was a young married woman in Welshpool, my husband – a keen fly fisherman – had been making some lead minnows and had cut two or three of his fingertips in the process. Some of the sand used in the moulds must have gone into the cuts but he did not mention this until his hand had swollen and an ominous red line was showing up his arm – blood poisoning was certainly indicated. This was on a Saturday, late afternoon, no chance of going to the local Doctor or seeing him until Monday. At that time we were living with my mother-in-law, a perfect dear incidently, and she had a friend who called now and then. She was a daughter of a famous blind Welsh preacher, one of a family of twelve. No doubt they treated most things themselves, a Doctor had to paid for in those days. When we showed her the swollen hand she asked 'Have you any fine oatmeal in the house?' Some was found and then she told me to mix some oatmeal with cold milk to a stiff paste – a bit thicker than one mixed mustard – and apply this on a clean rag, plenty of it to cover all the cuts and bind it up. That night my husband had a most uncomfortable time, he could feel this plaster as it hardened. The next morning when the bandage came off there was such an improvement that the remedy had worked.

Mrs. C. Mercer, Stafford

Cuts and Bleeding

When my mother was a little girl she cut her wrist badly, the bleeding could not be stopped. As there was no Doctor for some miles the assistance of one of the horsemen was called upon. He immediately on seeing the seriousness of the wound, ran to the stables, returning seconds later with a thick black cobweb taken from the rafters. It was laid in the cut and bound up, the bleeding stopped. My mother died forty years ago at the age of seventy-four, the cobweb that had staunched the flow of blood when she was but a child was still visible beneath the skin of her wrist.

T.J. Bowen, Essex

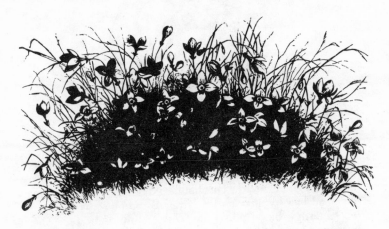

Boils and Constipation

In 1927 when I was in my late twenties, I was tormented by boils on my body, and although I cannot recall how it came about, nor who told me, I was advised to consume a nutmeg, grinding it first to a powder and mixing with water; now I am in my eighty-third year. Whether we like to admit it or not, in those far off days we were not overfed. Sunday dinner being the main meal of the week, the ritual on a Sunday morning was to line up for 'opening medicine', mostly in the shape of liquorice. This I remember was a yellow powder mixed with water – most horrible to take. The reason why this sticks in my mind so, it would seem that this was the price that had to be paid for having a meal.

E.J. Bourne, Essex

Fever

This was an old fashioned remedy applied to an uncle of mine in South Wales. As a child he was seriously ill for a number of days with a high temperature that would not break. The family were in an isolated community with no recourse to even the drugs available at that time, which would be about fifty years ago. His parents gathered a large number of earthworms from the garden and filled a man's woollen sock with them. The sock was then put around the child's neck and left there overnight. By the morning he was cool and the worms had dissolved into oil. I have heard this story from several sources in my family, and strange as it sounds, it is true.

Mrs. A. Mulcare, Berks.

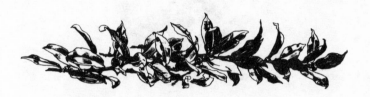

Septic Wounds, Boils and Carbuncles

Shortly after the introduction of penicillin into common usage (1950's) the squire of Credenhill village in Herefordshire had a nasty septic hand and one of his estate workers remarked upon it. 'Yes,' he was told 'I am putting penicillin on it.' 'Ah! yes,' was the reply, 'I am that grateful to that feller Alexander Fleming for discovering it.' 'How's that Tom?' 'Well Sir, its like this – you know those big hollow beech trees in Credenhill woods, with a lot of fungus around the bottoms?' 'Yes I know them.' 'Well sir, my mother, her mother and her mother before that always used to collect it up and mix it with Vaseline or any other grease and rub it on to any septic places, and it always cured them wonderfully. I have used it all my life, but I was never too happy about it, you know what I mean, fungus isn't too nice is it? But now I know what it is, and that it is all right, well I can use it anytime I like, can't I?'

Boils and carbuncles always seem to come in a series one after another. Onions won't cure them, but eating raw Spanish onions will stop the progression, they must have some effect on the blood stream. Laugh if you like, but the cure happens to work. One day the scrum half of English Steel Corporation Rugby Football Club in Sheffield started to miss matches because of boils on the back of his neck. The captain felt his loss and advised him to eat Spanish onions, but he bashfully refused on the grounds that he had only recently married and his wife might be put off him. A week later he was on the coach travelling for an away match with his wife, and they were *both* eating sandwiches with thick slices of onions as a filling . . . the boils had cleared.

H.A.B. Turner, Clwyd

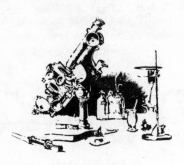

Hypertension

Writing to let you know of two people cured of hypertension using herbs. One was a cousin of mine, Steven Williams. The Doctor had told his sister Mrs. Minnie Williams that he had given up any hope of curing her brother, but she would not lose hope. She went to the countryside and picked the tender tips of stinging nettles, steeped them, slowly stewed them, strained them and bottled the juice. She gave a little wine-glassful a day to her brother, and after a few days he recovered. Another case was a school friend of Mother's, Cristobel Williams, not related to Steven. She also suffered with hypertension. Her doctor had also given up trying to cure her so she decided to go to London and get the advice and opinion from a specialist at Harley Street. He asked her all sorts of questions one being, 'Where are you from?' She told him. His advice: go back to Cornwall, pick tender tips of the stinging nettle that grow in abundance along most lanes, steep them, take a glass a day and you will be better in no time at all. His fee for this consultation? Twenty-five pounds. She did as the Harley Street specialist told her and lived happily for many years.

E.A. Barell, Essex

Toothache

I remember as a schoolboy in the 1920's, each dinner time Mother would give me a ha'penny or a penny to spend in the corner sweet shop on my way back to school. With this I would buy homemade treacle toffee (stickjaw we then called it). The months passed and inevitably my teeth became bad, and I suffered chronic toothache. So bad was the pain I attempted to pull these decaying teeth out with my fingers, only to break pieces from them and so make them worse. Mother would tip whisky into a spoon, I would dip my finger into the whisky and rub it around the affected gum. If this did not ease the pain I would tear off from under the bed mattress a six inch square piece of very old brown paper. Onto this mother would sprinkle a few drops of vinegar, into the centre. Then sprinkle pepper onto it, this was placed on my jaw and held in place by tying a woollen scarf around my head; this always relieved the pain, but left me with a bright red cheek.

Mr. E.F. Nash, Southampton

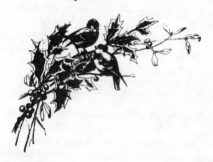

Scalds and Burns

When I was growing up in the 20's we always had a goose for Christmas Day dinner as a very dear aunt of mine – who fostered me for ten years – had a great faith in the healing balm of its grease for scalds and burns. The grease was saved and put into containers for when needed. I remember a neighbour who badly scalded her arm, quite possibly from water as she used to take in washing. On asking my aunt for advice, help was immediately given: the goose grease, on condition she let no-one else interfere. I think I am right – as this happened some sixty years ago – the neighbour's arm healed entirely and left no scarring.

Mrs. M. Bullick, Northumberland

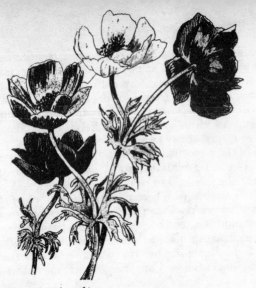

Sores and Bleeding

My mother always put ordinary white pepper on anything
that was bleeding, I mean of course minor sores. She used it
on me as a baby much to the horror of anyone who saw her,
but it does not hurt at all and does stop the bleeding.

Miss M. Bullick, Northumberland

Boils

About 1910, after serving in the Army for a number of years,
my father went to work on the railway in London, living in
lodgings. The change in living apparently affected him so
much, he came out in a crop of boils, all over his body. He
attended St. Mary's Hospital at Paddington for treatment, but
it did not do him any good; he became very weak and ill.
Feeling very down in the dumps, he went for a walk over
Hackney Marshes, where there were several gypsy families
living. One old lady saw him, asked what was wrong with
him, and on hearing his story and seeing his boils, she told
him to go to the gunsmith and buy a few pennyworth of
gunpowder. Get as much as would cover a sixpence, roll it in
a piece of butter and make a pill of it, and swallow it! Feeling
desperate, he did so, and lo and behold, the boils all erupted
and then cleared away and he never had another.

M. Sayers, Essex

Eczema, Skin Irritation and Ringworm

For the complaint eczema I have a soothing brew. This may not cure in all cases, but certainly curbs any irritation, and it is so simple to make. My father used it for years, and I have passed it on to endless numbers of people. It can also be used on animals suffering skin complaints. I collect an armful of chickweed, said to be the tastiest weed that can be eaten in salads. Wash well and place in bucket, pour on enough boiling water to just cover, leave overnight. Next day press down with washing tongs or potato masher and strain through colander; when settled strain through muslin or tea towel. Bottle and keep in refrigerator. I make enough to supply all my friends through the winter. I suffer a sore patch on my hand each summer, but this goes like magic when treated. Years ago my father had ringworm on his head, so treated it with the remedy. He went to the doctor who confirmed that it was ringworm but was surprised by the fact that it was dead, and asked father what he had treated it with. When told he was not too impressed.

Mrs. A. Birch, Hants.

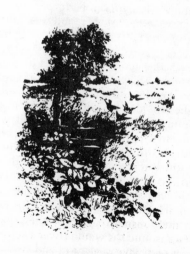

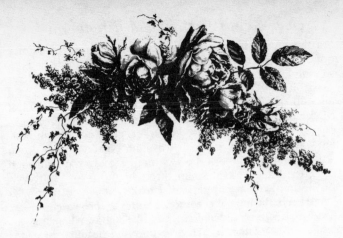

Rheumatic Fever

At the age of seven I became ill, the doctor told my mother I had rheumatic fever. For some months I lay in bed, the pains I suffered were terrible and to ease my boredom Father would, during the daytime, place my bed in the hallway so I was able to look out onto the road. The months passed, but still I was getting no better. One day an old gypsy came to the door selling her wares, Mother politely said she did not wish to purchase anything; the gypsy unperturbed by this queried as to what ailed me. Mother told her, and was quite taken aback by the old gypsy's reply 'Buy one of me vases my dear, and I will tell you a cure for that what ails yer youngin.' I have never known whether mother agreed just to get rid of her, or if it was because she believed what the old gypsy had said. For the next week she did as the old gypsy had told her. Three times a day she would grate salt from the block, enough to cover the bottom of a large roasting dish; it would then be placed in the oven to warm. This warmed salt was then put in equal amounts into a pair of socks and these my mother put on me. Each time they were taken off the salt that had been dry and warm was saturated with damp, one can only assume this dampness had been drawn from my feet. A week went by, Mother could see no results and in fact was thinking of stopping the treatment. Then one morning as she prepared breakfast, I walked into the room, the pains that had by then plagued me for nigh seven months had gone, it would seem the gypsy's salt cure had worked. At least that's what my mother and I believed, and still do.

D.E. Prince, Southampton

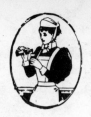

Abscess and Wasted Muscles

My mother was a great user of herbs and old remedies. One I remember was lily of the valley leaves steeped in boiling water, put into a muslin cloth then applied as a poultice on stubborn abscesses, bandaged and left overnight, repeated until relieved. My own son was a cripple for five and half years when he was young, with a rare bone disease; his limbs were very wasted, legs like sticks. We lived at that time in the country. The other side of the village lived a group of real Romanies in their caravans. We would lay our son on a spring bed placed on the lawn at the front of the cottage. The gypsies used to pass, one very old gypsy was called Grandmother Failn.

One summer I did at different times make some trousers and other things for her grandson because he protected my son at the village school from being pushed over by bigger boys. My son was in calipers. As Grandma Failn passed one day I mentioned to her that the lad's leg muscles were just wasted away, she said, 'You collect all the snails you can find, put them in an old clean container, and then crush them. Collect the frothy substance (green slime) that comes from them, free of shell of course, massage this frothy substance into the wasted flesh and muscle, twice a day.' Sounds revolting I know, but it feels like lanolin, even my own hands which were very work roughened, were like silk after a while. The difference in my son's legs was noticed by the orthopaedic specialist the next time he had to attend the hospital, he wanted to know what I had been doing to improve them so I said 'You will only laugh if I tell you.' Eventually I told him and his answer, without a laugh at all was, 'Grandmother Failn can work miracles.' This was over thirty-five years ago but thought you would be interested. I passed this cure onto two other people and it worked for them too.

Mrs. H.G. Doveless, Southampton

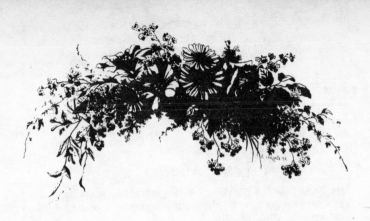

Cancer

My husband, after reading of your request for old cures in our local paper, was insistent that I wrote and told you a tale that happened to me as a young girl while in the service of a wealthy highland family. I was woken early and after a hurried breakfast I set to my chores, one of which was to ensure that the main hall and its entrance was kept clean. It was while cleaning the stone steps an old gypsy ambled up to me and asked to see the lady of the house. I pointed to the trade entrance, and explained that the mistress would not be very pleased to have him calling at the front of the house, and further to that she was very busy tending the master who was very ill. 'I knows that, that's reason I'm 'ere, now do as I ask an tell 'er I'm 'ere.' There was no need, for as I was about to get up the large door opened and the mistress appeared. 'Oh, do come in Mr. Jessop, thank goodness you were able to come.' The old gypsy gave me a knowing wink as he closed the door. Later in the kitchen, as I was about to have my midday meal the gypsy came in. 'I wants you tu fetch me a couple of sturdy thistles my gal.' The command was more of an order than request and as I had already given him cause earlier to report me to the mistress, I was not going to give him further reason. I put my meal back into the oven beside the range and left. The thistles he had asked me to fetch grew in abundance along the hedgerow of the road, so I was not gone long. Not knowing which part of the plant he required, after a little effort I was able to pull two out that had roots. I found out later that these were not needed, for when I gave them to him, he first removed the leaves and then chopped the roots and top off. Having left about four inches of stem from each thistle, these he placed into a saucepan containing about two pints of water. Before taking my meal from the oven I made a pot of tea, I asked if he would like one. 'Good idea, be a while 'fore this is ready.' About halfway through my meal curiosity got the better of me. 'What is that you are making Mr. Jessop?' 'That's my dear is a cure for cancer, only 'ope it aint bin left too late for yer master.' I, until then, had not known what illness ailed my employer and on hearing this I feared the worst, for never in my short life had I heard of anyone recovering from cancer. I pointed this out to the old gypsy, 'As wiv all 'erbal cures there ain't many that do know of 'um, tha's the problem, un' they thet do oney ave's a chance tu prove 'um when all they new fangled medicines 'as failed, by then its nearly always too late.' Six months after the gypsy called, the master was completely cured, and once again living a normal life. The reason I did not write before was that I did not wish to give false hope, but then as my husband pointed out supposing the old gypsy was right, and the thistle is able to cure or even prevent cancer?

Mrs. K.C. McDermott, Cornwall

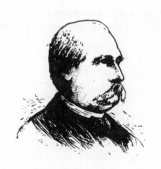

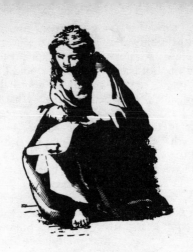